W0227820

Endometrial Cancer

Cancer Treatment and Research

WILLIAM L. MCGUIRE, *series editor*

Livingston R.B. (ed): Lung Cancer 1. 1981. ISBN 90–247–2394–9.
Humphrey G.B., Dehner L.P., Grindey G.B., Acton R.T. (eds): Pediatric Oncology 1. 1981.
ISBN 90–247–2408–2.
Decosse J.J., Sherlock P. (eds): Gastrointestinal Cancer 1. 1981. ISBN 90–247–2461–9.
Bennett J.M. (ed): Lymphomas 1, including Hodgkin's Disease. 1981. ISBN 90–247–2479–1.
Bloomfield C.D. (ed): Adult Leukemias 1. 1982. ISBN 90–247–2478–3.
Paulson D.F. (ed): Genitourinary Cancer 1. 1982. ISBN 90–247–2480–5.
Muggia F.M. (ed): Cancer Chemotherapy 1. ISBN 90–247–2713–8.
Humphrey G.B., Grindey G.B. (eds): Pancreatic Tumors in Children. 1982. ISBN 90–247–2702–2.
Costanzi J.J. (ed): Malignant Melanoma 1. 1983. ISBN 90–247–2706–5.
Griffiths C.T., Fuller A.F. (eds): Gynecologic Oncology. 1983. ISBN 0–89838–555–5.
Greco A.F. (ed): Biology and Management of Lung Cancer. 1983. ISBN 0–89838–554–7.
Walker M.D. (ed): Oncology of the Nervous System. 1983. ISBN 0–89838–567–9.
Higby D.J. (ed): Supportive Care in Cancer Therapy. 1983. ISBN 0–89838–569–5.
Herberman R.B. (ed): Basic and Clinical Tumor Immunology. 1983. ISBN 0–89838–579–2.
Baker L.H. (ed): Soft Tissue Sarcomas. 1983. ISBN 0–89838–584–9.
Bennett J.M. (ed): Controversies in the Management of Lymphomas. 1983. ISBN 0–89838–586–5.
Humphrey G.B., Grindey G.B. (eds): Adrenal and Endocrine Tumors in Children. 1983.
ISBN 0–89838–590–3.
DeCosse J.J., Sherlock P. (eds): Clinical Management of Gastrointestinal Cancer. 1983.
ISBN 0–89838–601–2.
Catalona W.J., Ratliff T.L. (eds): Urologic Oncology. 1983. ISBN 0–89838–628–4.
Santen R.J., Manni A. (eds): Diagnosis and Management of Endocrine-related Tumors. 1984.
ISBN 0–89838–636–5.
Costanzi J.J. (ed): Clinical Management of Malight Melanoma. 1984. ISBN 0–89838–656–X.
Wolf G.T. (ed): Head and Neck Oncology. 1984. ISBN 0–89838–657–8.
Alberts D.S., Surwit E.A. (eds): Ovarian Cancer. 1985. ISBN 0–89838–676–4.
Muggick P. (ed): Clinical Management of Gastrointestinal Cancer. 1983. ISBN 0–89838–601–2.
Pinedo H.M., Verweij J. (eds): Clinical Management of Soft Tissue Sarcomas. 1986. ISBN 0–89838–808–2.
Higby D.J. (ed): Issues in Supportive Care of Cancer Patients. 1986. ISBN 0–89838–816–3.
Surwit E.A., Alberts D.S. (eds): Cervix Cancer. 1987. ISBN 0–89838–822–8.
Jacobs C. (ed): Cancers of the Head and Neck. 1987. ISBN 0–89838–825–2.
MacDonald J.S. (ed): Gastrointestinal Oncology. 1987. ISBN 0–89838–829–5.
Ratliff T.L., Catalona W.J. (eds): Genitourinary Cancer. 1987. ISBN 0–89838–830–9.
Nathanson L. (ed): Basic and Clinical Aspects of Malignant Melanoma. 1987. ISBN 0–89838–856–2.
Muggia F.M. (ed): Concepts, Clinical Developments, and Therapeutic Advances in Cancer Chemotherapy.
1987. ISBN 0–89838–879–5.
Frankel A.E. (ed): Immunotoxins. 1988. ISBN 0–89838–984–4.
Bennett J.M., Foon K.A. (eds): Immunologic Approaches to the Classification and Management of
Lymphomas and Leukemias. 1988. ISBN 0–89838–355–2.
Osborne C.K. (ed): Endocrine Therapies in Breast and Prostate Cancer. 1988. ISBN 0–89838–365–X.
Lippman M.E., Dickson R. (eds): Breast Cancer: Cellular and Molecular Biology. 1988.
ISBN 0–89838–368–4.
Kamps W.A., Humphrey G.B., Poppema S. (eds): Hodgkin's Disease in Children: Controversies and
Current Practice. 1988. ISBN 0–89838–372–2.
Muggia F.M. (ed): Cancer Chemotherapy: Concepts, Clinical Investigations and Therapeutic Advances.   ·
1988. ISBN 0–89838–381–1.
Nathanson L. (ed): Malignant Melanoma: Biology, Diagnosis, and Therapy. 1988. ISBN 0–89838–384–6.
Pinedo H.M., Verweij J. (eds): Treatment of Soft Tissue Sarcomas. 1989. ISBN 0–89838–391–9.
Hansen H.H. (ed): Basic and Clinical Concepts of Lung Cancer. 1989. ISBN 0–7923–0153–6.
Lepor H., Ratliff T.L. (eds): Urologic Oncology. 1989. ISBN 0–7923–0161–7.
Benz C., Liu E. (eds): Oncogenes. 1989. ISBN 0–7923–0237–0.
Ozols R.F. (ed): Drug Resistance in Cancer Therapy. 1989. ISBN 0–7923–0244–3.
Surwit E.A., Alberts D.S. (eds): Endometrial Cancer. 1989. ISBN 0–7923–0286–9.

Endometrial Cancer

edited by

Earl A. Surwit. M.D.
Southern Arizona Surgical Oncology, Ltd.
Tucson, Arizona 85712

and

David S. Alberts, M.D.
University of Arizona
College of Medicine
Tucson, Arizona 85124

1989 **KLUWER ACADEMIC PUBLISHERS**
BOSTON / DORDRECHT / LONDON

Distributors

for North America: Kluwer Academic Publishers, 101 Philip Drive, Assinippi Park, Norwell, Massachusetts 02061 USA
for all other countries: Kluwer Academic Publishers Group, Distribution Centre, Post Office Box 322, 3300 AH Dordrecht, The Netherlands

Library of Congress Cataloging-in-Publication Data

Endometrial cancer/edited by Earl A. Surwit and David S. Alberts.
    p. cm. — (Cancer treatment and research)
  Includes bibliographies and index.
  ISBN-13: 978-1-4612-8210-5   e-ISBN-13: 978-1-4613-0867-6
  DOI: 10.1007/978-1-4613-0867-6

  1. Endometrium — Cancer. I. Surwit, Earl A. II. Alberts, David
S. (David Samuel), 1939–
  [DNLM: 1. Uterine Neoplasms. W1 CA693/WP 458 E551]
RC280.U8E48 1989
616.99′466 — dc20
DNLM/DLC
for Library of Congress   89-8183
                                              CIP

Copyright

© 1989 by Kluwer Academic Publishers

Softcover reprint of the hardcover 1st edition 1989

All rights reserved. No part of this publication may be reproduced, stored in a retrieval system or transmitted in any form or by any means, mechanical, photocopying, recording, or otherwise, without the prior written permission of the publisher, Kluwer Academic Publishers, 101 Philip Drive, Assinippi Park, Norwell, Massachusetts 02061, USA.

Dedication

We would like to dedicate this book to our children, Kara, Laura, and Rachel Surwit and Timothy and Sabrina Alberts, whose continued love and spirit have led to the success of our careers and to the energy responsible for the completion of this book. Such special children are truly a gift that we both will cherish forever.

Table of Contents

Preface

The incidence of endometrial cancer rose sharply in the United States in the early 1970s, paralleling changes in the use of postmenopausal estrogens by American women. A sizeable body of evidence supports the role of both excessive endogenous estrogen and exogenous estrogen in the etiology of endometrial cancer. There is growing evidence that inadequate progesterone has the opposite effect, in that progesterone supplementation of postmenopausal estrogen therapy reduces the incidence of endometrial cancer.

Despite this new awareness of the hormonal role that is played in carcinoma of the endometrium, the disease still plagues the oncologist. The general approach to carcinoma of the endometrium in the United States is that of primary surgical staging. This provides the maximum amount of information to best plan postoperative radiation therapy and/or chemotherapy for these patients. In general, patients who are considered candidates for surgical staging are those with advanced disease or high-risk stage I endometrial carcinoma. High-risk endometrial carcinoma is defined as those patients with moderately differentiated lesions with deep myometrial invasion, poorly differentiated carcinoma of the endometrium, and the high-risk histologies such as papillary carcinoma and clear-cell carcinomas. The surgical staging has extended in most institutions to patients with occult stage II carcinoma of the endometrium, i.e., cervical involvement (positive endocervical curettage), as this, too, provides the maximum amount of information for planning of postoperative radiotherapy and also spares those patients with stage I disease on final pathology from unnecessary radiation, unless it is indicated by other criteria.

The general approach to surgical staging of carcinoma of the endometrium is, in reality, quite straightforward and continues to include total abdominal hysterectomy and bilateral salpingo-oophorectomy with surgical staging, as noted above, for indicated cases, including pelvic and periaortic lymphadenectomy and pelvic cytology. Patients with papillary carcinomas of the endometrium tend to have a spread pattern similar to ovarian carcinoma, and, as a consequence, multiple intraperitoneal biopsies and cytologies along with omentectomy are included in the surgical staging for these patients.

Postoperative radiation therapy is then planned based on the information gleaned from the surgical staging. The approach taken by our group is that patients who have negative surgical staging and no myometrial invasion receive no further therapy. Patients with myometrial invasion that does not extend to within 5 mm of the serosal surface and who have negative surgical staging receive postoperative vaginal ovoids only.

However, those patients who have deep myometrial invasion, i.e., to within 5 mm of the serosal surface, and/or positive nodes, receive a combination of external radiation therapy and vaginal ovoids postoperatively. The external radiation therapy is tailored to the location of positive nodes.

The management of papillary carcinoma of the endometrium with positive surgical staging, particularly with intraperitoneal disease, is a difficult problem. There are some who advocate that these tumors are as sensitive as carcinomas of the ovary and should be treated with systemic platinum-based chemotherapy regimens. However, it is our current feeling that this is not the case, and we favor intraperitioneal chemotherapy with mitoxantrone for the patient with minimal residual disease, i.e., no single tumor nodule more than 5 mm in the peritoneal cavity, along with systemic cisplatin.

An important part of the surgical staging of all carcinomas of the endometrium is the obtaining of cytology at the time of entering the abdominal cavity, as this has also been proven to be an independent prognostic factor. Patients with positive cytology are treated aggressively with either intraperitioneal P–32 or whole-abdomen radiation therapy, depending on the additional findings at the time of surgical staging and the histological type of tumor.

Patients who are found to have adnexal involvement at the time of surgical staging are also treated aggressively with whole-abdomen radiotherapy, and there is significant evidence in the literature to support the efficacy of this approach.

The role of hormonal receptors in carcinoma of the endometrium has been well delineated, particularly in extensive in vivo animal models. Although there are difficulties to doing these studies, there would now appear to be clear rationale to suggest that the optimal hormonal approach to the treatment of patients with carcinoma of the endometrium would be sequential tamoxifen and progestational therapy. This is based on work that strongly suggests that tamoxifen is capable of turning on the progestational receptor, and it is well known that progestational agents turn off the progestational receptor, making these tumors no longer receptive to progestational therapy alone.

Unfortunately, the treatment of metastatic and/or recurrent carcinoma of the endometrium with cytotoxic chemotherapy remains relatively ineffective. Doxorubicin has been demonstrated to have the most significant activity as a single agent, with overall response rates approaching 40%. However, complete responses are rarely seen, and no significant improvement in survival has been demonstrated. Recently, both the North Central

Cancer Treatment Group and the Southwest Oncology Group have demonstrated significant activity for carboplatin as a single agent in the recurrent carcinoma of the endometrium. The overall response rate approximates 35%, and complete responses are seen in these patients. Unfortunately, to date no group-wide study has demonstrated an improved survival for multiagent chemotherapy in the treatment of carcinoma of the endometrium.

Despite the data demonstrating no improvement in survival for combination chemotherapy in this disease, commonly across the country patients are treated with a combination of doxorubicin and cisplatin. Currently the Gynecologic Oncology Group is doing a randomized prospective phase III trial comparing single-agent doxorubicin to doxorubicin and cisplatin to definitively answer this question.

Soon the Southwest Oncology Group will be investigating the combination of doxorubicin and carboplatin plus Granulocyte/Macrophage-Colony Stimulating Factor (GM-CSF) in a phase I/phase II setting. The use of GM-CSF should allow for an improved dose intensification of doxorubicin and carboplatin, which may lead to improved complete response rates. Hopefully this may lead to an improvement in results of combination chemotherapy for this disease.

In the treatment of patients with metastatic and/or recurrent carcinoma of the endometrium, it is important to recognize that the CA-125 tumor marker commonly utilized in ovarian cancer is frequently positive and may be very helpful in the management of these patients while they are on chemotherapy. Further development of monoclonal antibodies to specific endometrial carcinoma antigens could lead to a more accurate assessment of the extent of disease and to an improved therapeutic design for these patients.

List of contributors

ALBERTS, David S., Section of Hematology and Oncology, Department of Medicine, Arizona Health Sciences Center, University of Arizona, 1501 N. Campbell Avenue, Tucson AZ 85724, USA

BRENNER, MD, Dean E., Associate Professor of Internal Medicine and Pharmacology, University of Michigan Medical Ctr., Division of Hematology and Oncology, 4701 Upjohn Ctr., Ann Arbor, MI 48109-0504, USA

EINHORN, Nina, Associate Professor and Head, Dept of Gynecological Oncology, Radiumhemmet/Karolinska Hospital, Stockholm, Sweden

JONES, Charles M., III, Bowman Gray School of Medicine of Wake Forest University, Winston-Salem, NC 27103, USA

MORROW, C. Paul, Division of Gynecologic Oncology, LAC/USC Medical Center, Los Angeles CA 90033, USA

MORTEL, R., Department of Obstetrics and Gynecology, The Milton S. Hershey Medical Center, Pennsylvania State University, P.O. Box 850, Hershey PA 17033, USA

POTISH, Roger A., Associate Professor, Departments of Therapeutic Radiology and of Obstetrics and Gynecology, School of Medicine, University of Minnesota Hospital and Clinic, Box 494 UMHC, Harvard Street at E. River Road, Minneapolis MN 55455, USA

SALMON, Sydney E., Arizona Cancer Center, University of Arizona, 1501 N. Campbell Avenue, Tucson AZ 85724, USA

SATYASWAROOP, P.G., Department of Obstetrics and Gynecology, The Milton S. Hershey Medical Center, Pennsylvania State University, P.O. Box 850, Hershey PA 17033, USA

SUTTON, Gregory P., Associate Professor, Chief Gynecologic Oncology Department of Obstetrics and Gynecology, Indiana University School of Medicine, 926 W. Michigan Street, Indianapolis IN 46223, USA

THIGPEN, Tate, Professor of Medicine, Director of Division of Oncology, Department of Medicine, University of Mississippi School of Medicine, Jackson MS 39216, USA

VOIGT, Lynda F., The Fred Hutchinson Cancer Research Center, 1124 Columbia Street (W 108), Seattle, WA 98104, USA

WAIN, Gerard, Divison of Gynecologic Oncology, LAC/USC Medical Center, Los Angeles CA 90033, USA

WEISS, Noel S., The Fred Hutchinson Cancer Research Center, 1124 Columbia Street (W 108), Seattle, WA 98104, USA

WELANDER, Charles E., Bowman Gray School of Medicine of Wake Forest University, Winston-Salem, NC 27103, USA

ZAINO, R.J., Department of Pathology, The Milton S. Hershey Medical Center, Pennsylvania State University, P.O. Box 850, Hershey PA 17033, USA

Endometrial Cancer

1. Epidemiology of endometrial cancer

Lynda F. Voigt and Noel S. Weiss

Introduction

The incidence of endometrial cancer rose sharply in the United States in the early 1970s, paralleling changes in the use of postmenopausal estrogens by American women. A sizable body of evidence supports the role of both excessive endogenous estrogen and exogenous estrogen in the etiology of endometrial cancer. There is growing evidence that adequate progesterone has the opposite effect and that progestogen supplementation of postmenopausal estrogen therapy reduces the incidence of endometrial cancer.

Demographic correlates of the occurrence of endometrial cancer

Time

In the United States, the last two decades have seen large, rapid changes in the incidence of endometrial cancer. After a number of years of relative stability, the incidence in the early 1970s began to rise in most areas [1]. The increase in incidence was experienced primarily by women in the postmenopausal years and was generally greater in the western than in the eastern part of the country (Table 1). The increase shown in the table is actually a modest underestimate of the true one that occurred [2, 3]. The rate of hysterectomy (95 percent of which are performed for reasons other than cancer) rose rapidly during the same period, but the denominators of the cancer rates presented have not been corrected for this change [2, 4].

Some of the increase in incidence may be due to changes in the criteria used by pathologists for the diagnosis of endometrial carcinoma, and some is probably due to the increased incidence of estrogen-induced hyperplasia, a lesion whose morphology has many features in common with that of endometrial cancer and is sometimes labelled as such. Nonetheless, histologic reviews of cases diagnosed during the years of peak incidence, the mid-1970s, performed by pathologists using conservative criteria for the presence

E. Surwit and D. Alberts (eds.), ENDOMETRIAL CANCER. Copyright © 1989.
Kluwer Academic Publishers, Boston. All rights reserved.

Table 1. Annual incidence[a] of invasive carcinoma of the uterine corpus by age: Connecticut and Alameda County, California, 1960–1984.

Time period	Connecticut Age (years)		Alameda County[b] Age (years)	
	30–49	50–69	30–49	50–69
1960–64	15.4	66.5	11.0	70.6
1965–69	13.7	67.9	15.7	109.8
1970–71	11.6	77.1	17.0	135.6
1972–73	16.7	84.4	23.2	195.4
1974–75	14.7	99.4	18.5	186.7
1976–77	12.6	87.9	13.4	170.5
1978–79	14.6	95.3	6.1	119.1
1980–81	12.3	78.8	9.3	103.2
1982–83	9.4	77.7	8.5	87.5
1984	11.4	75.9	9.6	109.7

Data from Marrett LD, Elwood JM, Meigs JW, et al., 1978. Recent Trends in the Incidence and Mortality of Cancer of the Uterine Corpus in Connecticut. Gynecol Oncol 6:183; and Uterine Cancer Incidence Vol V #1, 1978, State of California, Department of Health; personal communications; and Surveillance, Epidemiology and End Results Program (SEER).
[a] Rate per 100,000 adjusted, within the broad age groups shown, to a uniform standard (ten-year age groups for Connecticut, five-year age groups for Alameda County).
[b] Whites only.

of cancer, found the incidence to be unequivocally greater than that of earlier years [5, 6].

In the later 1970s and early 1980s, the incidence of endometrial carcinoma in the United States declined (Tables 1, 2). In contrast to these rapid changes, the incidence during the past several decades outside of North America generally remained stable (Table 2) or increased to only a relatively small degree [7].

All the trends cited above run parallel to patterns of postmenopausal estrogen use. Although introduced into medical practice in the 1930s, estrogens were not widely taken by postmenopausal women in this country until the 1960s. Even then, consumption was greater in the western United States than in other regions [8], and outside of North American it generally remained uncommon [9]. Beginning in 1976, coincident with the documentation of the association between estrogens and endometrial cancer, there began a steady decline in the use of estrogens by American women, which lasted for several years; concomitant use of progestogen with estrogen has also increased [10–14].

Nationality

Even prior to the estrogen-stimulated increase in the incidence of corpus cancer, rates among United States' Caucasians were greater than rates among European women (Table 2) [15]. The incidence among black and

2

Table 2. Incidence of cancer of the uterine corpus in selected populations.

Continent	Country	Area	Race	'Truncated' incidence[a]		
				1969–72[b]	1973–77[c]	1978–82[d]
Africa	Nigeria	Ibadan	All	4.2	—	—
South America	Brazil	Sao Paulo	All	18.1	25.7	20.3
		Recife	All	4.1	—	8.9
	Columbia	Cali	All	11.3	9.8	9.2
North America	USA	Detroit	White	44.1	56.5	38.9
			Black	20.8	18.6	15.6
		New Mexico	Spanish	17.9	17.5	18.8
			Other White	39.0	53.7	30.9
			Am. Indian	11.4	9.2	9.7
Asia	India	Bombay	All	3.1	3.0	3.9
	Israel	All	Jews	22.9	21.4	16.6
			Non-Jews	3.1	1.7	6.0
	Japan	Miyagi	All	3.2	4.6	5.9
Europe	Norway	All	All	23.2	25.3	23.9
	U.K.	Oxford	All	20.7	22.7	18.2
	Yugoslavia	Slovenia	All	21.2	23.4	23.1
Oceania	USA	Hawaii	White	71.4	76.7	36.7
			Japanese	40.7	46.7	31.4
			Chinese	49.0	66.9	37.1
			Hawaiian	63.8	75.3	51.7
	New Zealand	All	Maori	58.1	33.4	31.5
			Non-Maori	22.8	24.3	17.6

[a] Annual rate per 100,000, ages 35–64, standardized to the age distribution of the World Standard Population.
[b] Waterhouse J, Muir C, Correa P, Powell J (eds), 1976. Cancer Incidence in Five Continents Vol III. Lyon: IARC Scientific Publications No. 15. Depending on population, rates apply to a part of the period 1969–1972.
[c] Waterhouse J, Muir C, Shanmugaratnam K, Powell J (eds), 1982. Cancer Incidence in Five Continents, Vol IV. Lyon: IARC Scientific Publications No. 42. Depending on population, rates apply to part of the period 1973–1977.
[d] Muir C, Waterhouse J, Mack T, Powell J, Whelan S (eds), 1987. Cancer Incidence in Five Continents, Vol V. Lyon: IARC Scientific Publications No. 88. Depending on population, rates apply to a part of the period 1978–1982.

Asian women in the United States also has been considerably above that of their counterparts in Africa and Asia. In Hawaii, Chinese and Japanese women have higher rates of corpus cancer than Caucasians in Europe. The high rate among Asian women in Hawaii was present in the early 1960s as well [16], arguing that factors other than exogenous estrogens have been responsible for it.

Age

The relation of the incidence of endometrial cancer to age depends, in part, on the degree of exposure of the postmenopausal female population to estrogens. When estrogen use is uncommon, the rates rise rapidly in late

3

reproductive life, peak in the 50s and 60s, and plateau or slightly decline in later life (Figure 1). In populations in which estrogen use is widespread among women in their 50s and 60s, the peak in incidence at these ages is accentuated.

Race

Maoris in New Zealand experience a rate of corpus cancer approximately twice that of non-Maoris (Table 2); the incidence among the latter is comparable to that of European whites. The high rate among Maoris is not due to an unusually high incidence of corpus cancer that is non-endometrial in nature [F. Foster, personal communication]. Hawaiian women also have a relatively high incidence of corpus cancer (Table 2), so it may be that some feature of their shared Polynesian background is responsible.

In other parts of the world, the incidence of corpus cancer among Caucasians exceeds that among women of other races (Table 2). However, the white/black difference in the United States depends on age (Figure 1), as it is not present in women before the age of 40 nor beyond age 70. The similarity of rates at older ages is due, at least in part, to the inclusion of non endometrial tumors, whose incidence rises rapidly with age and is higher in blacks than in whites [17].

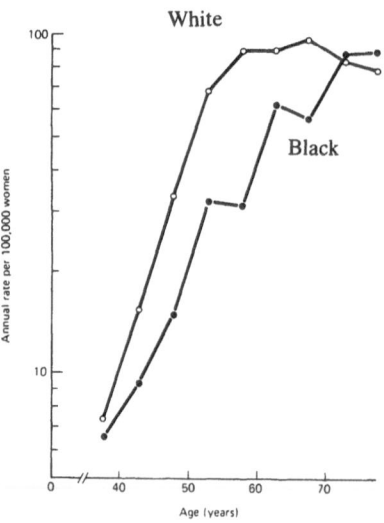

Figure 1. Incidence of cancer of the uterine corpus, by age and race: US third national cancer survey, 1969–1971. (From the Third National Cancer Survey: Incidence Data. Monograph 41, March 1975.

Risk factors

Hormonal

Endogenous estrogens. Cellular proliferation is a prerequisite for carcinogenesis [18]; unchecked proliferation can lead to malignant transformation [19]. Since estrogens are the primary stimulants of endometrial proliferation, it follows that their presence may be a necessary condition for the development of at least some endometrial carcinomas. The data available support such a role for estrogens.

1. In the presence of estrogen-secreting ovarian tumors, the prevalence of endometrial carcinoma at the time of oophorectomy ranges from 6 to 21% [20–23]. Even allowing for possible biases in the selection of cases and in the use of liberal criteria in determining the presence of uterine cancer, it is likely that the observed frequency of this second primary tumor is considerably greater than expected.

2. Elevated levels of estrogens can arise from an excessive production of other hormones that can be converted to estrogens. For example, women who have polycystic ovaries and amenorrhea or oligomenorrhea (the polycystic ovary syndrome) secrete abnormally large quantities of androstenedione. This is aromatized peripherally, resulting in persistent estrone levels characteristic of the peak of the normal ovulatory cycle [24]. An unusually high proportion of young women with endometrial cancer [25, 26] and endometrial hyperplasia [27] have polycystic ovaries.

Several groups of women with the polycystic ovary syndrome have been followed with no cases of endometrial cancer found [28, 29], but as the expected incidence in these young women was exceedingly low, the presence of an increased relative risk could not be ruled out.

3. Obesity has been shown to increase the amount of endogenous estrogen available to target tissues through three mechanisms: differential estrogen metabolism, increased conversion of androstenedione to estrogen, and decreased levels of sex hormone binding globulin. Obesity decreases the metabolism of estrogen via the C–2 hydroxylation pathway [30], a pathway that produces an estrogen metabolic that is relatively inactive. Peripheral conversion of androstenedione to estrone is the primary source of estrogens in postmenopausal women and is believed to occur primarily in adipose tissue. The rate of this conversion is greater in obese women than in lean women [31–33]. Finally, levels of sex hormone binding globulin, which are influential in determining levels of biologically available estrogen, are inversely related to weight [34].

A consistent finding in studies of endometrial cancer is that cases are more likely to be overweight than controls, in both pre- and postmenopausal women [35–47]; the relative risk associated with being overweight has been estimated to be two to 20 times greater, depending in part on the criterion used to measure it.

Lack of endogenous progesterone. Progesterone is the only endogenous progestogen of biological importance. The surge of progesterone secretion which begins just prior to ovulation each month in the premenopausal women, arrests endometrial proliferation, promotes secretory differentiation of the endometrium, and initiates endometrial sloughing in the absence of fertilization [48–53]. These actions would be expected to discourage the development of cancer, since cell differentiation alone can arrest or reverse neoplastic cellular transformation [19]. Epidemiologic evidence is compatible with a protective effect of progesterone.

1. Endometrial cancer is rare in premenopausal women. Its peak incidence occurs during the first or second decade after the menopause (Figure 1), a time of life in which limited estrogen production continues (through peripheral conversion of adrenal androgens) but in which there is no cyclic progesterone production and minimal peripheral production of progesterone.

2. Women with the polycystic ovary syndrome, who are at increased risk of endometrial cancer, are characterized not only by an excessive production of estrogen but also by the absence of cyclic progesterone secretion [26, 54, 55].

3. The increased risk of endometrial cancer in obese women may be related to decreased progesterone levels as well as, or instead of, a hyperestrogenic state. A study of six obese oligomenorrheic premenopausal women and ten nonobese controls found consistently subnormal levels of serum progesterone, even though the luteal phase lasted at least ten days [56]. Estrogen levels did not differ between the two groups.

4. A retrospective cohort study of 1,270 women with chronic anovulatory syndrome found three times the expected number of cases of subsequent invasive endometrial cancer during the 14,499 woman-years of follow-up [57]. Anovulatory cycles are associated with impaired progesterone secretion [58], indicating that this increased risk may be related to lack of endogenous progesterone.

5. The increased risk of endometrial cancer seen in women who have undergone a relatively late menopause [36–41, 59] may relate to perimenopausal progesterone levels that provide inadequate opposition to continuing estrogen production. The perimenopausal period is characterized by an increasing number of anovulatory cycles and diminished luteal phase function [60, 61], resulting in decreased progesterone production [58].

Exogenous estrogens. For several decades estrogens have been taken by women during and after menopause, and early on it was appreciated that these women develop adenomatous hyperplasia of the uterus more commonly than do other women [62]. Endometrial biopsies have shown conversion of normal endometrium to cystic or adenomatous hyperplasia in 12 to 44% of women who received either cyclic or continuous estrogens after six to 12 months of use [63–65]. A case control study of adenomatous endometrial hyperplasia found a sixfold increase in risk associated with estrogen replacement therapy [66]. The credibility of this association is strengthened by the fact that some hyperplastic lesions regress when estrogen is discontinued [67]. Adenomatous and cystic hyperplasia probably represent an early stage in the development of endometrial carcinoma, as they frequently coexist with endometrial cancer in estrogen users and have been observed to precede the appearance of carcinoma [68–70]. A follow-up study of 170 women with untreated hyperplasia found that 1.6% of the women with simple hyperplasia and 23% of the women with atypical hyperplasia developed endometrial cancer [71].

A listing of published case-control studies which have examined estrogen use in relation to endometrial cancer incidence is shown in Table 3. Excluded from the list are those studies whose design led to a falsely low measure of the magnitude of the association: (1) studies that failed to exclude from the control group women who had undergone hysterectomy, and (2) studies that included as controls women with estrogen-related conditions (e.g., postmenopausal vaginal bleeding). All but two of the 20 studies shown found a greater proportion of women with endometrial cancer had taken estrogens than had controls. In addition, in every one of the case-control studies it was found that risk increased with increasing duration of use [40–43, 46, 72–75, 77–83]. In general, the estimates of relative risk associated with long duration of use of estrogens, e.g., greater than five years, were in greater agreement than those for all durations combined.

Apart from duration, the size of an estrogen user's excess risk may be influenced by other features of her use.

Time since first use. All studies which reported data on elapsed time between first use of estrogen and development of endometrial cancer found that the estrogen user's risk exceeded that of the nonusers by the sixth year of use [40–43, 46, 78, 85]. The time at which the excess risk is first present is not clear. Some have found it within the first year of use [58, 72], others by the fifth year of use [73, 75], and one not until the sixth year [46].

Time since last use. All ten studies that examined this question found a fall in the excess risk once estrogen use ceased (Table 4). In two studies there remained no residual excess after two drug-free years had elapsed [46, 83]. One found risk was still elevated after two years [84]. Two found the risk persisted for at least five years [78, 81], while one study found increased risk after ten drug-free years [82].

Type of estrogen. All listed studies of users of conjugated estrogens have found them to be at increased risk of developing endometrial cancer; the studies in Finland and Sweden, however, found no increased risk to estrogen users as a whole [83, 86]. Of all the studies in the United States that examined the effect of other estrogens (e.g., stilbestrol or ethinyl estradiol), nine of the 12 observed a positive relationship. Percutaneous

7

Table 3: Summary of published articles on menopausal estrogens and the incidence of endometrial cancer.

First author	Reference	Area of residence or hospitalization	Cases			Relative risk (ever vs. never used)
			Years of diagnosis	Number	Estrogen users (%)	
Antunes (1979)	72	Baltimore, MD	1973–77	344	19.0	4.9
Buring (1986)	81	Boston, MA	1970–75	188	38.8	2.4
Gray (1977)	73	Louisville, KY	1947–76	205	22.0	3.0
Hoogerlund (1978)	74	Madison, WI	1960–74	587	18.0	2.3
Hulka (1980)	46	Chapel Hill, NC	1970–76	186	33.0	1.4
Jelovsek (1980)	75	Durham, NC	1940–75	431	12.0	2.4
Jick (1979)	76	Seattle, WA	1975–77	67	90.0	11.3
Kelsey (1982)	43	New Haven, CT	1977–79	148	40.5	2.2
LaVecchia (1984)	42	Milan, Italy	1979–83	283	25.0	1.6
McDonald (1977)	77	Olmsted County, MN	1945–74	106	23.0	2.3
Mack (1976)	84	Southern CA	1971–75	63	83.0	8.0
Pettersson (1986)	83	Uppsala Region, Sweden	1980–81	250	20.1	1.2
Salmi (1980)	86	Turku, Finland	1970–76	282	33.0	0.6
Shapiro (1980)	78	13 North American hospitals	1976–79	149	40.0	3.9
Shapiro (1985)	82	Eight United States, hospitals and Ontario, Canada	1976–82	425	31.0	3.5
Smith (1975)	97	Seattle, WA	1960–72	317	48.0	4.5
Spengler (1981)	40	Toronto, Canada	1977	88	45.0	3.2
Stavraky (1981)	41	London, Canada	1976–78	206	47.0	4.8
Weiss (1979)	85	Seattle-Tacoma, WA	1975–76	322	78.0	7.0
Ziel (1975, 1976)	79, 80	Los Angeles, CA	1970–74	94	57.0	7.6

Table 4: Summary of published articles on time since last estrogen use and risk of endometrial cancer.

First author	Reference	Interval	Relative risk*
Buring	81	≥5 years	4.5
Hulka	46	≥20 months	1.0
Mack	84	≥2 years	3.4
Pettersson	83	≥2 years	0.9
Shapiro**	78	≥5 years	2.6
Shapiro	82	≥10 years	1.9
Stavraky	41	≥1 year	1.4
Weiss	85	≥8 years	3.0

* Referent group = Women who never used estrogens.
** Users included only women with five or more years of use.

estradiol has also been reported to induce proliferative endometrium [87], and an increased risk of endometrial cancer has also been reported among users of vaginal hormone creams [43].

Dose. In the range commonly prescribed, 0.3 mg to 1.25 mg per day of conjugated estrogens (or the equivalent amount of other estrogens), the risk of endometrial cancer is increased for all doses and appears to rise with increasing dose.

Periodic interruption of use. Many women who take estrogens are instructed to discontinue them for one week each month. Of the eight studies that compared this method to that of continuous exposure, two found risks highest from continuous use, two from cyclic use, and four found no difference [41, 46, 72, 77, 78, 81, 84, 85]. The fact that the incidence of endometrial hyperplasia is no different in groups of women on the two regimens [63] also argues that there is little to distinguish them in terms of subsequent cancer risk.

Two prospective studies that monitored postmenopausal estrogen users over time for cancer incidence have been reported [88, 89] with results roughly similar to those of the case-control studies.

Other studies that monitored women receiving estrogens for reasons other than amelioration of menopausal symptoms provide additional information about the long-term effects of estrogen supplementation. Young women with gonadal agenesis who received stilbestrol (a synthetic, nonsteroidal estrogen) for prolonged periods had an unusually high incidence of endometrial cancer [90]. Although there have been no studies of cancer incidence among untreated women with this condition, there is no biologic reason to suspect gonadal dysgenesis, per se, as an etiologic factor. In a group of patients with breast cancer who had received estrogenic hormones (primarily stilbestrol) for treatment of their disease, the subsequent incidence of endometrial cancer was about twice that expected on the basis of rates in other breast cancer patients [91].

Although several studies have reported an increased risk associated with estrogen use for invasive and higher grade cancers [43, 46, 72, 82, 85], the highest risks are seen in the less invasive and more highly differentiated tumors [43, 81, 82, 85]. This is reflected in a more favorable survival experience among estrogen-using cases [92–95].

There are reasons to believe that all of the following are responsible for the particularly strong association of estrogen use with less invasive tumors than those of nonusers [96]:

1. some cases of estrogen-related adenomatous hyperplasia are falsely labelled as early endometrial cancer (see previous discussion).
2. On the average, endometrial cancer is detected earlier in estrogen users than in nonusers.
3. Endometrial tumors that arise in the presence of high estrogen levels tend to be biologically less aggressive than other endometrial tumors.

The results of studies of endometrial cancer in relation to the use of noncontraceptive estrogens, taken together with: (1) the correlation of time trends in the incidence of endometrial cancer and estrogen use in the United States; (2) the growth-stimulating effect of exogenous estrogens on endometrial tissue, which can lead to the development of premalignant lesions; and (3) the role that endogenous estrogens are known to play in the etiology of this cancer, argue strongly that exogenous estrogens are a cause of endometrial cancer. Endometrial neoplasms that arise from the action of these hormones do so relatively quickly, often in less than five years. In many women, this adverse effect of estrogens is 'reversible,' in that, within a year or two, stopping the use of the drug reduces the size of the excess risk. Thus it appears that exogenous estrogens act at a relatively late stage in the development of endometrial cancer, most likely through the stimulation of growth of cells with malignant potential.

Lack of exogenous progestogens. Exogenous progestogens mimic the actions of luteal progesterone in promoting differentiation of endometrial glands and arresting endometrial proliferation. These beneficial effects persist even when low-dose progestogens are given continuously in combination with estrogens with no endometrial sloughing [98–100]. Estrogen-stimulated hyperplasias have reverted to normal endometrium after administration of progestogens [65, 105]. Prospective studies have found a duration-related decrease in incidence of hyperplasia in women on a progestogen-estrogen regimen, compared to women receiving only estrogens [101]. Ten to thirteen days of progestogen have been found by most studies to induce secretory changes comparable to those of the secretory menstrual cycle, using progestin dosages as low as .35 mg per day of norethindrone [49, 51, 102, 103]. Whitehead et al. found hyperplasia occurred in 3–4% of women on a seven day progestogen cycle [50]. Thom found reduced hyperplasia in women on five to ten days use of progestogen (compared to estrogen-only users) and no hyperplasia in women on more than ten days of use [105]. Patterson also found no hyperplasia after ten days of progestogen in conjunction with oral estrogen [106]. Sturdee and Thom found no hyperplasia after ten to 13 days of progestogens, when used in conjunction with either oral or subcutaneous estrogen [64, 105].

Women who are exposed to exogenous progestogens through use of combination oral contraceptives have about one-half the risk of endometrial cancer as do nonusers (Table 5). On the other hand, women who used Oracon, a sequential preparation that employed dimethisterone (a weak progestogen with a large dose of a potent estrogen, ethinyl estradiol), were found to be at an increased risk of endometrial cancer [44, 107, 108]. While two other studies found no excess risk associated with the use of Oracon [43, 109], their subjects were all diagnosed after Oracon had been taken off the market, so the influence of 'current' use could not be evaluated. The risk associated with the use of other sequential oral contraceptives remains unclear (Table 5), partially due to the small numbers of women who reported use of these OCs.

Most studies of the relationship of combination oral contraceptives to endometrial cancer reported decreasing risk as duration of OC use increased [43, 44, 59, 109–111]; two studies found no difference according to duration of use [112, 113]. The interval since the last use of OCs was generally not associated with any change in endometrial cancer risk, although the number of users was too small to adequately address this issue [44, 107, 109, 110, 113]; one study reported a lower risk for current users compared to past users [111].

Epidemiological data on the effect of progestogen supplementation of postmenopausal estrogens on the risk of endometrial cancer have been sparse. One study of 43 women who developed endometrial cancer after estrogen replacement therapy found that the risk among women who had progestogen supplementation for at least half of the time the estrogens were used was one-third the risk of the women who used estrogen alone [88]. A study conducted at a military hospital over a nine year period accrued 31 cases of endometrial cancer over 27,243 woman-years of observation. The estrogen-progestogen users had a significantly lower crude incidence of endometrial cancer (49 per 100,000) than either the unopposed estrogen users (391 per 100,000) or the nonhormone users (246 per 100,000) [115]. Hunt, however, reported an increased incidence of endometrial cancer both among recipients of estrogen-progestogen and recipients of estrogen-only replacement therapy (twelve cases occured, half of whom had progestogen supplementation, compared to an expected occurrence of 4.3 cases) [89]. In the latter study, the monthly duration of progestogen therapy was shorter than that of most women taking this hormone today.

Events of reproductive life

The data regarding the relationship of age at menarche to endometrial cancer is mixed, with some studies reporting an earlier menarche among cases than among controls [42, 43, 93, 110], whereas others have reported

Table 5. Summary of published articles on oral contraceptives to the risk of endometrial cancer.

First author	Ref	Study area	Year of diagnosis	Ages of subjects (years)	Number of cases	% OC users among cases	Type of OC	RR
Armstrong (1988)	113	Multisites in 7 developing countries	1979–85	25–59	140	10.0	Combination only	0.5
						0.7	Any sequential	1.2
CDC and steroid hormone study (1983)	110	Multisites, USA	1980–81	20–54	187	17.0	Combination only	0.5
						2.6	Any sequential	2.1
Henderson (1983)	44	Los Angeles County, CA	1972–79	<45	127	39.0	Combination	0.5
						8.7	Any sequential	1.9
						4.7	Oracon	2.1
Hulka (1982)	111	North Carolina	1970–76	30–60	79	6.3	Combination	0.4
Kaufman (1980)	109	Multisites, USA and Canada	1976–79	<60	154	10.5	Combination	0.5
						1.0	Any sequential	0.7
						0.6	Oracon	1.0
Kelsey (1982)	43	Connecticut	1977–79	45–55	37	16.0	Any	0.6
LaVecchia (1986)	114	Milan, Italy	1979–85	<60	283	4.1	Combination	0.5
Petterson (1986)	59	Uppsala Region, Sweden	1980–81	34–60	108	11.1	Any	0.5
Trapido (1983)	112	Boston, MA	1970–76	25–57	98	20.4	Any	1.4
Weiss (1980)	107	King and Pierce Counties, WA	1975–77	35–54	117	15.0	Combination	0.5*
							Sequential	
						5.5	Oracon	7.3*
						0.9	Other	0.3

* One or more years of use.

no difference [36, 40, 59, 84]. In contrast to findings on breast cancer, most studies [36, 38, 93, 43], though not all [39], have found age at first birth to be unrelated to the incidence of endometrial cancer.

A woman's probability of developing endometrial cancer is inversely related to the number of children she has borne [36–40, 43, 44, 59]. In addition to nulliparity, impaired fertility (three or more years of unsuccessfully attempting pregnancy or physician diagnosed infertility) has also been associated with an increased risk of endometrial cancer [44, 110].

Women who experience menopause at a relatively late age are at greater risk of endometrial cancer than are other women [36–42, 59]. The presence of menstrual cycles into a woman's fifties indicates the continued presence of ovarian-produced estrogens and may also reflect inadequate opposing progesterone.

Other risk factors

Abnormal glucose tolerance and diabetes mellitus. Although the relationship between diabetes and endometrial cancer has been commonly investigated and long cited, there remains some doubt as to its nature and magnitude. A recent study by Pettersson found no difference in fasting blood glucose among endometrial cancer cases and controls [45]. However, the relevance of a woman's glucose tolerance after the diagnosis of cancer to that prior to the inception of cancer is uncertain. A case-control study which attempted to take account of these problems, and also controlled for an important confounding variable, body weight, found an increased frequency of antecedent diabetes among endometrial cancer patients [37]; another found only a slight increase [43]. However, four others observed no increase [40, 41, 45, 111]. Finally, two studies that mointored the occurrence of cancer among cohorts of diabetics found neither the incidene of nor the mortality from endometrial cancer to be increased [116, 117]. However, both studies lacked statistical power to detect a relatively small excess. In summary, though abnormal glucose tolerance might predispose a woman to the development of endometrial cancer, the question is by no means settled.

Elevated arterial pressure. The study of the role of high blood pressure in the etiology of endometrial cancer is plagued by the same kinds of difficulties present for elevated blood sugar: inaccuracies in the retrospective assessment of hypertension, lack of standardized blood pressure measurements in routine clinical records, and the presence of important confounding variables which require control. At the present time, it is unclear whether any relationship exists. Three studies that controlled for age and weight estimated the endometrial cancer risk in women with a history of hypertension to be 30 to 100% greater than that among normotensives [37, 38, 45]. A third study also found a higher proportion of cases than controls to have high blood pressure, but there was an excess of women among the cases with low blood pressure as well [36]. Four additional studies found no association at all [40, 41, 43, 111].

Gall bladder disease. After taking exposure to exogenous estrogens into account, two studies [38, 84] found a greater proportion of women with prior gall bladder disease among endometrial cancer cases than among controls. It is possible that this association is due to the association of endogenous estrogens to both conditions.

Radiation exposure. Studies that have monitored the incidence of cancer in women receiving therapeutic pelvic radiation have mixed results. Three reported an increased risk for uterine cancer [118–120], and three reported no increased risk [121–123]. One study found an increased incidence only for uterine sarcomas and not for other uterine malignancies [124]. However, the condition which led to the therapeutic radiation could be confounding the results of these studies. There does not seem to be an increased risk from total body irradiation, since the mortality of uterine corpus cancer has not shown an increase among Japanese atomic bomb survivors [125].

Cigarette smoking. Every case-control study of endometrial cancer that has ascertained cigarette smoking behavior has noted a lower proportion of smokers among cases than among controls (Table 6). The negative association has been particularly strong in recent smokers, which would be predicted if smoking were to exert an effect by interfering in some way with the action of estrogens in endometrial carcinogenesis. The observed case/control difference has generally been somewhat greater in postmenopausal than

Table 6. Influence of menopausal status on the association between cigarette smoking and endometrial cancer.

| Author | Reference | Comparison | Relative risk in: | |
			Premenopausal women	Postmenopausal women
Weiss	38	Ever-smoker vs nonsmoker	0.5	0.4
Lesko	128	≥25 cigarettes/day vs nonsmoker	0.9	0.5
Stockwell	129	Current smoker vs nonsmoker	1.0*	0.8**
Franks	130	Current smoker vs nonsmoker	0.7	0.5
Lawrence	47	Current smoker vs nonsmoker	0.6	0.6
Levi	131	Current smoker vs nonsmoker	0.5	0.4

* Women <50 years of age.
** Women ≥50 years of age.

14

in premenopausal women. Thus if cigarette smoking does prevent some women from developing endometrial cancer, it is likely to do so in ways other than by reducing ovarian production of estrogens. The most likely explanation seems to be differential estrogen metabolism among smokers, favoring the 2–hydoxyestrone pathway, which produces a metabolite of low estrogenic activity [126]. This explanation is strengthened by the findings of a clinical trial in which postmenopausal women were randomized to various hormonal regimens or placebo. The smokers in every treatment group, but no in the placebo group, showed decreased levels of serum estrogen [127].

Genetic factors. In a study conducted in a population in which estrogen use was uncommon, there was little if any tendency for endometrial cancer to occur in families more often than would have been expected by chance [36]. Kelsey, however, found an increased risk of endometrial cancer in women reporting endometrial or ovarian cancer in a mother or sister [43]. The absence of an increased risk for women with a family history of breast cancer in that study argues against recall bias.

Future directions

The evidence to date supports the role of estrogens, whether the hormones are endogenously-derived or exogenously-dervied, in the development of endometrial carcinoma. It seems likely that the role of progestogens, derived from whatever source, is the opposite. Knowledge of these effects will allow, through the judicious use (or nonuse) or these hormones, the prevention of many cases of endometrial cancer. Nonetheless, there will continue to be many women who produce relatively great amounts of estrogen and/ or small amounts of progesterone. Many others will continue to use 'unopposed' noncontraceptive estrogen preparations, because of concern with short-term and potential long-term adverse cardiovascular effects of supplemental progestogens. One important thrust of future research will be to determine the amount of progestogen that maximizes the protection against endometrial cancer while minimizing any negative impact on the cardiovascular system. An additional important issue is further identification of characteristics and exposures that interact with gonadal hormones to produce or prevent the disease; the knowledge of such modifying factors can assist an individual women and her physician in making a more informed decision regarding hormone replacement therapy.

References

1. Weiss NS, Szekely DR, Austin DF, 1976. Increasing incidence of endometrial cancer in the United States. N Engl J Med 294:1259–1262.
2. Lyon JL, Gardner JW, 1977. The rising frequency of hysterectomy: Its effect on uterine cancer rates. Am J Epidemiol 105:439–443.

3. Howe HL, 1984. Age-specific hysterectomy and oophorectomy prevalance rates and the risks for cancer of the reproductive system. Am J Public Health 74:560–563.
4. Koepsell TD, Weiss NS, Thompson DJ, et al., 1980. Prevalence of prior hysterectomy in the Seattle-Tacoma area. Am J Public Health 70:40–47.
5. Szekely DR, Weiss NS, Schweid AI, 1978. The incidence of endometrial carcinoma in King Country, Washington: A standarized histologic review. JNCI 60:985–989.
6. Gordon J, Regan JW, Finkel WD, et al., 1977. Estrogen and endometrial carcinoma: An independent pathology review supporting original risk estimate. N Engl J Med 297:570–571.
7. Pagel J, Bock JE, 1984. Endometrial cancer. Dan Med Bull 31:333–345.
8. Jick H, Walker AM, Rothman KJ, 1980. The epidemic of endometrial cancer: A commentary. Am J Public Health 70:264–267.
9. Doll R, Kinlen LJ, Skegg DCG, 1976. Incidence of endometrial carcinoma. Br Med J 1:1071–1072.
10. Austin DF, Rode KM, 1982. The decreasing incidence of endometrial cancer: Public health implications. Am J Public Health 72:65–68.
11. Standeven M, Criqui MH, Klauber MR, et al., 1986. Correlates of change in postmenopausal estrogen use in a population-based study. Am J Epidemiol 124:268–274.
12. Gruber JS, Luciani CT, 1986. Physicians changing postmenopausal sex hormone prescribing regimens. In Advances in Cancer Control: Health Care Financing and Research. Alan R. Liss, pp. 325–335.
13. Ross RK, Paganini–Hill A, Roy S. et al., 1988. Past and present preferred prescribing practices of hormone replacement therapy among Los Angeles gynecologists: Possible implications for public health. Am J Public Health 78:516–519.
14. Kennedy DL, Baum C, Forbes MB, 1985. Noncontraceptive estrogens and progestins: Use patterns over time. Obstet Gynecol 65:441–446.
15. Waterhouse J, Muri C, Correa P, et al. (eds), 1976. Cancer Incidence in Five Continents, Vol III. Lyon: IARC Scientific Publications No 15.
16. Doll R, Muir CS, Waterhouse J. (eds), 1970. Cancer Incidence in Five Continents, Vol II. Geneva: UICC.
17. Harlow BL, Weiss NS, Lofton S, 1986. The epidemiology of sarcomas of the uterus. JNCI 76:399–402.
18. Ryser HJP, 1971. Chemical carcinogenesis. N Engl. J Med 285:721–734.
19. Pitot C, 1986. Fundamentals of oncology. New York: Dekker.
20. Diddle AW, 1952. Granulosa and theca cell ovarian tumors: Prognosis. Cancer 5:215–228.
21. Larson JA, 1954. Estrogens and endometrial cancer. Obstet Gynecol 3:551–572.
22. Salerno LJ, 1962. Feminizing mesenchymomas of the ovary — An analysis of 28 granulosa-theca cell tumors and their relationship to coexistent carcinoma. Am J Obstet Gynecol 84:731–738.
23. Gusberg SB, Kardon P, 1971. Proliferative endometrial response to theca-granulosa cell tumors. Am J Obstet Gynecol 111:633–643.
24. Siiteri PK, MacDonald PC, 1973. The role of extra-glandular estrogen in human endocrinology. Handbook of Physiology 2:615.
25. Dockerty MB, Lovelady SB, Foust GT, Jr, 1951. Carcinoma of the corpus uteri in young women. Am J Obstet Gynecol 61:966–981.
26. Farhi DC, Nosanchuk J, Silverberg SG, 1986. Endometrial adenocarcinoma in women under 25 years of age. Obstet Gynecol 68:741–745.
27. Charmlian DL, Taylor HB, 1970. Endometrial hyperplasia in young women. Obstet Gynecol 36:659–666.
28. Stein IF, 1958. The Stein–Leventhal syndrome — A curable form of sterility. N Engl J Med 259:420–423.
29. Leventhal ML, 1958. The Stein–Leventhal syndrome. Am J Obstet Gynecol 76:825–836.
30. Schneider J, Bradlow HL, Strain G, et al., 1983. Effects of obesity on estradiol meta-

16

bolism: Decreased formation of nonuterotropic metabolites. J Clin Endocrinol Metab 56:973–978.

31. MacDonald PC, Siiteri PK, 1974. The relationship between the extraglandular production of estrone and the occurrence of endometrial neoplasia. Gynecol Oncol 2:259–263.

32. McDonald PC, Edman CD, Hemsell DL, et al., 1978. Effect of obesity on conversion of plasma androstenedione to estrone in postmenopausal women with and without endometrial cancer. Am J Obstet Gynecol 130:448–455.

33. Edman CD, MacDonald PC, 1978. Effect of obesity on conversion of plasma androstenedione to estrone in ovulatory and anovulatory young women. Am J Obstet Gynecol 130:456–461.

34. Davidson BJ, Gambone JC, Lagasse LD, et al., 1981. Free estradiol in postmenopausal women with and without endometrial cancer. J Clin Endocrinol Metab 52:404–408.

35. Damon A, 1960. Host factors in cancer of the breast and uterine cervix and corpus. JNCI 24:483–516.

36. Wynder EL, Escher GC, Mantel N, 1966. An epidemiological investigation of cancer of the endometrium. Cancer 19:489–520.

37. Elwood JM, Cole P, Rothman KJ, et al., 1977. Endometrial cancer: Fertility and other factors. JNCI 59:1055–1060.

38. Weiss NS, Farewell VT, Szekely DR, et al., 1980. Oestrogens and endometrial cancer: Effect of other risk factors on the association. Maturitas 2:185–190.

39. LaVecchia C, Franceshi S, Gallus G, et al., 1982. Oestrogens and obesity as risk factors for endometrial cancer in Italy. Int J Epidemiol 11:120–126.

40. Spengler RF, Clarke EA, Woolever A, et al., 1981. Exogenous estrogens and endometrial cancer: A case-control study and assessment of potential bias. Am J Epidemiol 114:497–506.

41. Stavraky KM, Collins JA, Donner A, et al., 1981. A Comparison of estrogen use by women with endometrial cancer, gynecologic disorders, and other illnesses. Am J Obstet Gynecol 141:547–555.

42. LaVecchia C, Franceschi S, DeCarli A, et al., 1984. Risk factors for endometrial cancer at different ages. JNCI 73:667–671.

43. Kelsey JL, Livolsi VA, Holford TR, et al., 1982. A case-control study of cancer of the endometrium. Am J Epidemiol 116:333–342.

44. Henderson BE, Casagrande JT, Pike MC, et al., 1983. The epidemiology of endometrial cancer in young women. Br J Cancer 47:749–756.

45. Petterson B, Adami HO, Bergstrom R, 1985. Obesity, hypertension and diabetes as risk factors for endometrial cancer. In Risk Factors for Endometrial Carcinoma. Uppsala: Acta Universitatis Upsaliensis.

46. Hulka BS, Fowler WC, Kaufman DG, et al., 1980. Estrogen and endometrial cancer: Cases and two control groups from North Carolina. Am J Obstet Gynecol 137:91–101.

47. Lawrence C, Tessaro I, Durerian S, et al., 1987. Smoking, body weight and early stage endometrial cancer. Cancer 59:1665–1669.

48. Hammond CB, Jelovsek FR, Lee KL, Creasman WT, Parker RT, 1979. Effects of long-term replacement therapy: I. metabolic effects. Am J Obstet Gynecol 133:525–536.

49. Siddle NC, Townsend PT, Young O, et al., 1982. Dose-dependent effects of synthetic progestins on the biochemistry of the estrogenized post-menopausal endometrium. Acta Obstet Gynecol Scand Supp 106:17–22.

50. Whitehead MI, King RJB, Mcqueen J, et al., 1979. Endometrial histology and biochemistry in climacteric women during oestrogen and oestrogen/progestogen therapy. J Roy Soc Med 72:322–327.

51. King RJB, Whitehead MI, 1983. Estrogen and progestin effects on epithelium and stroma from pre- and postmenopausal endometria: Application to clinical studies of the climacteric syndrome. In Steroids and Endometrial Cancer (Jasonni VM, ed). New York: Raven Press.

52. King RJB, Dyer G, Collins WP, et al., 1980. Intracellular estradiol, estrone, and estrogen

17

receptor levels in endometria from postmenopausal women receiving estrogens and progestins. J Steroid Biochem 13:377–382.

53. Leeson TS, Roland LC, 1981. Histology, Fourth Edition. Philadelphia: WB Saunders.

54. Lucas WE, 1974. Causal relationships between endocrine-metabolic variables in patients
with endometrial carcinoma. Obstet Gynecol Surv 29:507–528.

55. Yen SSC, 1980. The polycystic ovary syndrome. Clinical Endocrinology (Oxf) 12:177–
208.

56. Sherman BM, Korenman SG, 1974. Measurement of serum LH, FSH, estradiol and
progesterone in disorders of the human menstrual cycle: The inadequate luteal phase. J
Clin Endocrinol Metab 39:145–149.

57. Coulam CB, Annegers JF, Kranz JS, 1983. Chronic anovulation syndrome and associated
neoplasia. Obstet and Gynecol 61:403–407.

58. Johansson EDB, 1984. The sterile menstrual cycle. Acta Obstet Gynecol Scand Suppl
123:147–150.

59. Pettersson B, Adami HO, Berstrom R, et al., 1986. Menstrual span — A time limited risk
factor for endometrial cancer. Acta Obstet Gynecol Scand 65:247–255.

60. Sherman BM, 1987. Endocrinologic and menstrual alterations. In Menopause: Physiology
and Pharmacology (Mishell DR, ed). Chicago: Year Book Medical Publishers, Inc., pp.
41–51.

61. Benson RC, 1980. Handbook of Obstetrics and Gynecology. Los Altos, CA: Lange
Medical Publications.

62. Gusberg SB, 1947. Precursors of corpus carcinoma estrogens and adenomatous hyperplasia. Am J Obstet Gynecol 54:905–927.

63. Schiff I, Sela HK, Cramer D, 1982. Endometrial hyperplasia in women on cyclic or
continuous estrogen regimens. Fertil Steril 37:79–82.

64. Sturdee DW, Wade–Evans T, Paterson MEL, et al., 1978. Relations between bleeding
pattern, endometrial histology and oestrogen treatment in menopausal women. Br Med J
1:1575–1577.

65. Whitehead MI, McQueen RJ, Beard RJ, et al., 1977. The effects of cyclical oestrogen
therapy and sequential oestrogen/progestogen therapy on the endometrium of postmenopausal women. Acta Obstet Gynecol Scand Suppl 65:91–101.

66. Krieger N, Marrett LD, Clarke AE, et al., 1986. Risk factors for adenomatous endometrial hyperplasia: A case-control study. Am J Epidemiol 123:291–301.

67. Kistner RW, 1973. Endometrial alterations associated with estrogen and estrogen-
progestin combinations. In The Uterus (Norris HJ, Hertig AT, Abell MR, eds). Balti-
more: Williams and Wilkins.

68. Gusberg SB, Hall RE, 1961. Precursors of corpus cancer III. The appearance of cancer of
the endometrium in estrogenically conditioned patients. Obstet Gynecol 17:397–412.

69. Pettersson B, Adami HO, Lindgren A, et al., 1985. Endometrial polyps and hyperplasia
as risk factors for endometrial carcinoma. Acta Obstet Gynecol Scand 64:653–659.

70. Deligdisch L, Holinka CF, 1987. Endometrial carcinoma: Two Diseases? Cancer Detect
Prev 10:237–246.

71. Kurman RJ, Kaminski PF, Norris HJ, 1985. The behavior of endometrial hyperplasia: A
long term study of 'untreated' hyperplasia in 170 patients. Cancer 56:403–412.

72. Antunes CMF, Stolley PD, Rosenshein NB, et al., 1979. Endometrial cancer and estrogen
use: Report of a large case-control study. N Engl J Med 300:9–13.

73. Gray, LA, Christopherson WM, Hoover RN, 1977. Estrogens and endometrial carcinoma. Obstet Gynecol 49:385–389.

74. Hoogerland DL, Buchler DA, Crowley JJ, Carr WF. Estrogen use — risk of endometrial
carcinoma. Gynecol Oncol 6:451–458.

75. Jelovsek FR, Hammond CB, Woodard BH, et al., 1980. Risk of exogenous estrogen
therapy and endometrial cancer. Am J Obstet Gynecol 137:85–91.

76. Jick H, Watkins RN, Hunter JR, et al., 1979. Replacement estrogens and endometrial
cancer. N Engl J Med 300:218–222.

18

77. McDonald TW, Annegers JF, O'Fallon WM, et al., 1977. Exogenous estrogen and endometrial carcinoma: Case-control and incidence study. Am J Obstet Gynecol 127:572–580.
78. Shapiro S, Kaufman DW, Slone D, et al., 1980. Recent and past use of conjugated estrogens in relation to adenocarcinoma of the endometrium. N Engl J Med 303:485–489.
79. Ziel HK, Finkle WD, 1975. Increased risk of endometrial carcinoma among users of conjuated estrogens. N Engl J Med 293:1167–1170.
80. Ziel HK, Finkle WD, 1976. Association of estrone with the development of endometrial carcinoma. Am J Obstet Gynecol 124:735–740.
81. Buring JE, Bain CJ, Ehrmann RL, 1986. Conjugated estrogen use and risk of endometrial cancer. Am J Epidemiol 124:434–441.
82. Shapiro S, Kelly JP, Rosenberg L, et al., 1985. Risk of localized and widespread endometrial cancer in relation to recent and discontinued use of conjugated estrogens. N Engl J Med 313:969–972.
83. Pettersson B, Adami HO, Persson I, et al., 1986. Climacteric symptoms and estrogen replacement therapy in women with endometrial carcinoma. Acta obstet Gynecol Scand 65:81–87.
84. Mack TM, Pike MC, Henderson BE, et al., 1976. Estrogens and endometrial cancer in a retirement community. N Engl J Med 294:1262–1267.
85. Weiss NS, Szekely DR, English DR, Schweid AI, 1979. Endometrial cancer in relation to patterns of menopausal estrogen use. JAMA 242:261–264.
86. Salmi T, 1980. Endometrial carcinoma risk factors, with special reference to the use of oestrogens. Acta Endocrinol 233:37–43.
87. Holst J, Cajander S, von Schoultz B, 1983. Cellular morphometric analysis of the postmenopausal endometrium during treatment with percutaneous estradiol–17B with and without oral gestagen. Acta Obstet Gynecol Scand 62:267–270.
88. Persson IR, Adami HO, Eklund G, et al., 1986. The risk of endometrial neoplasia and treatment with estrogens and estrogen-progestogen combinations. Acta Obstet Gynecol Scand 65:211–217.
89. Hunt K, Vessey M, McPherson K, et al., 1987. Long-term surveillance of mortality and cancer incidence in women receiving hormone replacement therapy. Br J Obstet Gynaecol 94:620–635.
90. Cutler BS, Forbes AP, Ingersoll FM, et al., 1972. Endometrial carcinoma after stilbesterol therapy in gonadal dysgenesis. N Engl J Med 287:628–631.
91. Hoover R, Fraumeni JF, Everson R, et al., 1976. Cancer of the uterine corpus after hormonal treatment for breast cancer. Lancet 1:885–887.
92. Robboy SJ, Bradley R, 1979. Changing trends and prognostic features in endometrial cancer associated with exogenous estrogen therapy. Obstet Gynecol 54:269–277.
93. Elwood JM, Boyes DA, 1980. Clinical and pathological features and survival of endometrial cancer patients in relation to prior use of estrogens. Gynecol Oncol 10:173–187.
94. Collins J, Allen LH, Donner A, et al., 1980. Oestrogen use and survival in endometrial cancer. Lancet 2:961–963.
95. Chu J, Schweid AI, Weiss NS, 1982. Survival among women with endometrial cancer: A comparison of estrogen users and nonusers. Am J Obstet Gynecol 143:569–573.
96. Weiss NS, 1978. Noncontraceptive estrogens and abnormalities of endometrial proliferation. Ann Intern Med 88:410–412.
97. Smith DC, Prentice R, Thompson DJ, et al., 1975. Association of exogenous estrogen and endometrial carcinoma. N Engl J Med 293:1164–1167.
98. Staland B, 1985. Continuous treatment with a combination of estrogen and gestagen — A way of avoiding endometrial stimulation. Acta Obstet Gynecol Scand Suppl 130:29–35.
99. Mattsson L, Samsioe G, 1985. Estrogen-progestogen replacement in climacteric women, particularly as regards a new type of continuous regimen. Acta Obstet Gynecol Supp 130:53–58.
100. Magos AL, Brincat, M, Dowd T, et al., 1985. Amenorrhoea and endometrial atrophy

19

following continuous oral oestrogen and progestogen therapy in post-menopausal women. Obstet Gynecol 65:496–499.

101. Whitehead MI, 1978. The Effects of oestrogens and progestogens on the post-menopausal endometrium. Maturitas 1:87–96.
102. Whitehead MI, Townsend PT, Pryse–Davies J, 1981. Effects of estrogens and progestins on the biochemistry and morphology of the postmenopausal endometrium. N Engl J Med 305:1599–1605.
103. King RJB, Whitehead MR, 1986. Assessment of the potency of orally administered progestins in women. Fertil Steril 46:1062–1066.
104. Whitehead MI, Townsend PT, Pryse–Davies J, et al., 1982. Effects of various types of progestogens on the postmenopausal endometrium. J Reprod Med 27:539–548.
105. Thom MH, White PJ, Williams RM, et al., 1979. Prevention and treatment of endometrial disease in climacteric women receiving oestrogen therapy. Lancet 2:455–457.
106. Paterson MEL, Wade–Evans T, Sturdee DW, et al., 1980. Endometrial disease after treatment with oestrogens and progestogens in the climacteric. Br Med J 280:822–824.
107. Weiss NS, Sayvetz T, 1980. Incidence of endometrial cancer in relation to the use of oral contraceptives. N Engl J Med 302:551–554.
108. Silverberg SG, Makowski EL, Roche WD, 1977. Endometrial carcinoma in women under 40 years of age. Cancer 39:592–598.
109. Kaufman DW, Shapiro S, Slone D, et al., 1980. Decreased risk of endometrial cancer among oral-contraceptive users. N Engl J Med 303:1045–1047.
110. The Centers for Disease Control, 1983. Oral contraceptive use and the risk of endometrial cancer. JAMA 249:1600–1604.
111. Hulka BS, Chambless LE, Daufman DG, et al., 1982. Protection against endometrial carcinoma by combination-product oral contraceptives. JAMA 247:475–477.
112. Trapido EJ, 1983. A prospective cohort study of oral contraceptives and cancer of the endometrium. Int J Epidemiol 12:297–300.
113. Armstrong BK, Ray RM, Thomas DB, 1988. Endometrial cancer and combined oral contraceptives. Int J Epidemiol 17:263–269.
114. Lavecchia C, DeCarli A, Fasoli M, et al., 1986. Oral contraceptives and cancers of the breast and of the female genital tract. Interim results from a case-control study. Br J Cancer 54:311–317.
115. Gambrell RD, Jr, 1986. Prevention of endometrial cancer with progestogens. Maturitas 8:159–168.
116. Kessler II, 1970. Cancer mortality among diabetics. JNCI 44:673–680.
117. Ragozzino M, Melson LJ, Chu C–P, et al., 1982. Subsequent cancer risk in the incidence cohort of Rochester, Minnesota residents with diabetes mellitus. J Chronic Dis 35:13–19.
118. Corscaden JA, Fertig JW, Gusberg SB, 1946. Carcinoma subsequent to the radiotherapeutic menopause. Am J Obstet Gynecol 51:1–12.
119. Stander RW, 1957. Irradiation castration: A follow-up study of results in benign pelvic disease. Obstet Gynecol 10:223–229.
120. Wagoner JK, 1984. Leukemia and other malignancies following radiation therapy for gynecologic disorders. In Radiation Carcinogenesis: Epidemiology and Biological Significance (Boice JD, Fraumeni JF, Jr eds). New York: Raven Press, pp. 153–159.
121. Hunter RM, Ludwick V, Motley JF, et al., 1954. The use of radium in the treatment of benign lesions of the uterus: A critical twenty-year survey. Am J Obstet Gynecol 67:121–129.
122. Doll R, Smith PG, 1968. The long-term effects of X irradiation in patients treated for metropathia haemorrhagica. Br J Radiol 41:362–368.
123. Boice JD, Day NE, Andersen A, et al., 1984. Cancer risk following radiotherapy of cervical cancer: A preliminary report. In Radiation Carcinogeneses: Epidemiology and Biological Significance (Boice JD, Fraumeni JF, eds). New York: Raven Press.
124. Czesnin K, Wronkowski Z, 1978. Second malignancies of the irradiated area in patients treated for uterine cervix cancer. Gynecol Oncol 6:309–315.

125. Kato H, Schull WJ, 1982. Studies of the mortality of A-bomb survivors, 7. Mortality, 1950–1978: Part 1. Cancer mortality. Rad Res 90:395–432.
126. Michnovicz JJ, Hershcopf RJ, Naganuma H, et al., 1986. Increase of 2–hydroxylation of estradiol as a possible mechanism for the anti-estrogenic effect of cigarette smoking. N Engl J Med 315:1305–1309.
127. Jensen J, Christiansen C, Rodbro P, 1985. Cigarette smoking, serum estrogens, and bone loss during hormone-replacement therapy early after menopause. N Engl J Med 313:973–975.
128. Lesko SM, Rosenberg L, Kaufman DW, et al., 1985. Cigarette smoking and the risk of endometrial cancer. N Engl J Med 313:593–596.
129. Stockwell HG, Lyman GH, 1987. Cigarette smoking and the risk of female reproductive cancer. AM J Obstet Gynecol 157:35–40.
130. Franks AL, Kendrick JS, Tyler CW, et al., 1987.
131. Levi F, LaVecchia C, DeCarli A, 1987. Cigarette smoking and the risk of endometrial cancer. Eur J Cancer Clin Oncol 23:1025–1029.
132. Waterhouse J, Muri C, Shanmugaratnam K, Powell J. (eds), 1982. Cancer Incidence in Five Continents, Vol IV. Lyon: IARC Scientific Publications No 42.

2. Surgical management of endometrial cancer

Gerard Wain and C. Paul Morrow

Introduction

One of the basic principles of clinical oncology is recognition of the extent of disease at the time of presentation and tailoring of therapy to encompass the full extent of the malignant process. Such a process, when applied to individual patients, must take into account the extent of clinically detectable disease, the problems of spread, and the presumed preexisting clinically occult disease. Only then can adequate therapy be offered.

The application of such a broad principle to carcinoma of the endometrium represents a challenge to the gynecologic oncologist. Carcinoma of the endometrium is the most common gynecologic malignancy, and it is estimated that approximately 35,000 new cases will be diagnosed in 1987 [1]. Using the widely accepted staging system of the International Federation of Gynecologists and Obstetricians (FIGO) (Table 1), approximately 80% will present as Stage I. While it is true that the survival for advanced stages is consistently poorer, thus giving some prognostic value to FIGO staging, the fact that most patients present with 'early' disease reduces the prognostic and therapeutic value of this staging system. Furthermore, within Stage I disease there are widely variant survival rates reported. Although a commonly accepted absolute five-year survival is around 90% [2, 3], the 1985 Annual Report of FIGO reports a much lower corrected survival of about 75% [4]. Still others, looking at specific poor prognostic groups within Stage I, report very much lower survival figures; for example, Aalders et al. [5] reported a 40% five-year survival for clinical Stage I disease with surgically diagnosed adnexal extension, and Chambers et al. [6] reported a 72.9% five-year survival for Stage I patients with histology showing poorly differentiated adenocarcinoma (Grade 3).

These figures demand a process of risk analysis in each patient with early stage endometrial adenocarcinoma, so that appropriate diagnostic and therapeutic steps can be taken to correctly assess and treat the full extent of the malignancy. An important contribution to this process has been made by the recently published surgical staging data of the Gynecologic Oncology Group (GOG) [7], and the application of these data to individual patients will be described.

E. Surwit and D. Alberts (eds.), ENDOMETRIAL CANCER. Copyright © 1989.
Kluwer Academic Publishers, Boston. All rights reserved.

Table 1. FIGO clinical staging for carcinoma of the corpus uteri.

Stage 0	Atypical hyperplasia or carcinoma in situ. Histologic findings suspicious of malignancy. Cases of stage 0 should not be included in any therapeutic statistics.
Stage I	The carcinoma is confined to the corpus.
Stage Ia	The length of the uterine cavity is 8 cm or less.
Stage Ib	The length of the uterine cavity is more than 8 cm.

Stage I cases should be subgrouped with regard to the histologic type of the adenocarcinoma as follows:

G1-highly differentiated adenomatous carcinoma.

G2-moderately differentiated adenomatous carcinoma with partly solid areas.

G3-predominantly solid or entirely undifferentiated carcinoma.

Stage II	The carcinoma has involved the corpus and the cervix, but has not extended outside the uterus.
Stage III	The carcinoma has extended outside the uterus, but not outside the true pelvis.
Stage IV	The carcinoma has extended outside the true pelvis or has obviously involved the mucosa of the bladder or rectum. A bullous edema as such does not permit a case to be allotted to Stage IV.
Stage IVa	Spread of the growth to adjacent organs.
Stage IVb	Spread of the growth to distant organs.

Clinical staging

The FIGO staging system is a clinical staging system and takes into account uterine size, histological grade, and clinincally detectable metastases or extension into neighboring or distant sites. The staging system allows those examinations and procedures that are presumed to be universally available: palpation, inspection, colposcopy, hysteroscopy, fractional curettage, roentgen examination of the lungs and skeleton, and intravenous pyelography [8]. The Cancer Committee of FIGO does not allow information obtained from other diagnostic procedures to be included in the staging process: specifically lymphography, arteriography, venography, hysterography, ultrasound, laparoscopy, computerized tomography (CT), or magnetic resonance imaging (MRI). In particular, information gained at the time of surgery or subsequent pathological examination cannot change an allocated staging.

Physical examination and fractional curettage are the mainstays in assigning a clinical stage. The supraclavicular and inguinal nodes are palpated and the abdomen examined for masses, ascites, enlarged liver, and umbilical metastases. The vulva is rarely involved by endometrial cancer, but the anterior, distal vagina is a fairly common site for metastases and qualifies a case for Stage III allocation. These suburethral metastases are usually submucosal and, therefore, readily overlooked. Bimanual rectovaginal examination determines the uterine size, shape, mobility and position, the character of the parametrial tissues, and the condition of the adnexae. On vaginal examination, any target lesion of the cervix or vagina is biopsied and the uterine cavity is sounded. The endocervix and isthmus are curetted before the endometrium (fractional curettage), and separate endocervical and endometrial specimens are sent to the laboratory. FIGO allows a chest

Table 2. Prognostic factors in endometrial carcinoma.

Patient factors:	Age
	Ethnic origin
	Health
	Previous radiation exposure
Tumor extent:	Clinical stage
	Cervical involvement
	Adnexal involvement
	Peritoneal cytology
	Uterine size
Histopathological features:	Histologic type and grade
	Nuclear grade
	Myometrial invasion
	Vascular space invasion
	Hormone receptor content
Treatment factors:	quality of surgical and radiation therapy

x-ray and intravenous pyelogram (IVP) to complete staging. Using these principles, the distribution by stage of disease was 80.8, 10.7, 4.2, and 4.2 per cent for Stages I, II, III, and IV respectively in a 1981 nationwide accumulation reported by Wharton [9].

While FIGO staging may have broad prognostic implications (Table 2) and may be useful for comparative statistical purposes, the practicing gynecologist need not feel similarly restricted in the use of diagnostic procedures that may help in the preliminary assessment of each patient and the formation of a rational plan of treatment.

Hysteroscopy and hysterography have been employed to determine the configuration of the tumor, its proximity to the isthmus, and endocervical involvement. We have not incorporated these studies into our staging workup because of the potential for forcing tumor particles into the fallopian tubes or uterine vascular spaces. A recent report, however, found tumor size and lower uterine or cervical extension to be important prognostic indications of the lymph node metastasis and suggested hysteroscopy as a preoperative means of assessing these factors [10].

CT scanning and MRI provide valuable information about the lungs, retroperitoneum, peritoneum, and liver parenchyma, which cannot be obtained by clinical means, particularly in the obese patient (Figure 1). These studies should be used selectively. Hricak [11] compared staging by MRI with surgical-pathologic staging in 51 patients with an overall staging accuracy of 92%. Limitations of the technique, however, include the inability to distinguish adenomatous hyperplasia or blood clots from endometrial carcinoma. Most significantly, such noninvasive techniques do not preclude the need for surgical management of most patients.

Radionucleotide scanning of the liver or bone should not be a routine part of the workup. Mettler [12] showed these to be positive in only 2% and 3% respectively, and suggests that symptomatology, advanced disease or

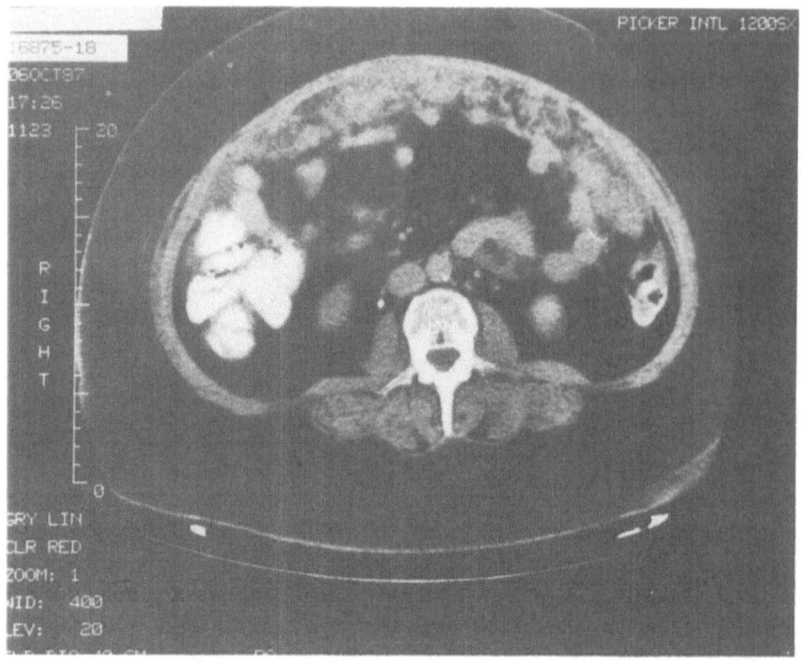

Figure 1. CT scan of a patient with clinical Stage III endometrial carcinoma showing ascites and an omental cake. Subsequent laparotomy confirmed widespread intraperitoneal disease.

abnormal liver function tests, should be used to select patients for these studies.

Pelvic ultrasound may provide useful information preoperatively in the assessment of ascites, pelvic masses, or coexistent uterine pathology, such as fibroids. This information cannot be used for staging, however, and again does not eliminate the need for surgical exploration.

Consideration must be given, finally, to the possible presence of other malignancies in this group of patients, who are clearly at risk epidemiologically. Wharton found that 525 of 7,220 patients (7.7%) had second primary tumors at the time of diagnosis: particularly breast, colon, and ovarian cancer [9]. In Nori's series [13], 12 of 300 patients (4%) with early stage disease died of other cancers, including colon, bladder, breast, and lymphoma. These facts highlight the need for thorough physical examination, breast examination, and examination of stool for occult blood. Mammography, barium studies, and sigmoidoscopy should be performed when specifically indicated.

The tumor marker CA–125 has proven to be of value in monitoring response and relapse in endometrial carcinoma and should be measured preoperatively [14]. Elevation of CA–125 should direct a search for metastatic disease, as such elevation has some correlation with advanced disease [15].

Table 3. Grade, depth of invasion and pelvic node metastasis.

| Depth of invasion | Grade | | | | | |
| | G1 (N=180) | | G2 (N=288) | | G3 (N=153) | |
	Pelvic	Aortic	Pelvic	Aortic	Pelvic	Aortic
Endometrium only (86)	0 (0%)	0 (0%)	1 (3%)	1 (3%)	0 (0%)	0 (0%)
Inner (N=281)	3 (3%)	1 (1%)	7 (5%)	5 (4%)	5 (9%)	2 (4%)
Middle (N=115)	0 (0%)	1 (5%)	6 (9%)	0 (0%)	1 (4%)	0 (0%)
Deep (N=139)	2 (11%)	1 (6%)	11 (19%)	8 (14%)	22 (34%)	15 (23%)

Adapted from Creasman et al. [7]. Numbers in brackets refer to percentages of each subgroup.

Table 4. Comparison of five-year survival of Stage II endometrial carcinoma patients with clinically occult or gross involvement.

| Study | Occult | | Gross | |
	N	Survival (%)	N	Survival (%)
Larson et al. 1987 [34]	48	65	10	70
Kinsella et al. 1980 [35]	37	95	18	44
Homesley, Boronow, & Lewis 1977 [36]	61	61	23	48
Onsrud et al. 1982 [37]	86	82	10	60
Bruckman et al. 1978 [38]	28	93	12	66
Boronow 1973 [39]	14	61	19	58

Adapted from Morrow [33]

Prognostic factors

The generally good survival and the preponderance of early stage disease in patients with endometrial cancer has lead to a certain complacency in attitude toward the disease, resulting in significant undertreatment for some patients and, paradoxically, overtreatment in others. In an attempt to avoid each of these problems, attention is now directed to specific risk factors in each patients, which correlate with the degree of local spread, metastases, chance of recurrence, and likelihood of survival. Using this information, therapy can be designed on an individual basis, depending on the presence or absence of these factors. More than 15 factors of importance have been reported in the literature (Table 2). The recently published data from the groupwide Gynecologic Oncology Group surgical pathological staging series [7] have given impetus to a process of risk-factor analysis for each patient, helping the clinician to devise the optimal, individualized treatment plan that will minimize overtreatment as well as undertreatment (Table 5).

Prior to discussing such a process and its application to the surgical management of these patients, we will briefly consider some of the major prognostic factors.

27

Uterine size

Although incorporated in FIGO staging, uterine size or cavity length appears to have a variable correlation with prognosis. Combining the results of Frick et al. [16], DePalo et al. [17], and Kauppila et al. [18], the five-year survival rate for FIGO Stage IA cases is 86.4% (591/684) compared to 75.3% (530/704) for Stage IB cases. Others, however, have reported no significant survival difference for these substages [19, 20]. The obvious fact that uterine enlargement need not reflect tumor size very accurately should restrain the clinician from overestimating the prognostic signficance of this factor.

Age and menopausal stages

The GOG data shows no increased risk of nodal metastasis between pre-menopausal and post-menopausal patients. Aalders et al. [19] showed that death and recurrence rates increase with age: women older than 60 years show significantly higher rates than women under 60 years. The distribution of histological grade was comparable between the two groups, but myometrial invasion was significantly greater in the older age group. Chambers [6] suggested that being greater than 65 years of age and being of older age at menopause are significant but he does not specify the age level at menopause at which significance can be placed. In the report from Memorial-Sloan Kettering [13], premenopausal patients had a better overall prognosis than postmenopausal patients (95% versus 82%), and a multivariant analysis demonstrated that patients who are less than 55 years of age have a better outcome compared to those who are older than 55 years.

The suggestion of two pathogenic varieties of endometrial carcinoma on the basis of the presence or absence of various epidemiological features (e.g., obesity, diabetes, hypertension, and anovulation) [21] may help explain some of the inconsistencies in published reports of survival data in young patients [22]. Awareness of a higher incidence of such poor prognostic factors in a subgroup of young patients without these epidemiologic features may help identify a subgroup at higher risk. Such a statement, however, rests to a large extent on unsubstantiated supposition.

Histology

The literature agrees that tumor differentiation is very important in predicting extrauterine spread, nodal metastasis, recurrence, and survival, with poorly differentiated lesions carrying a very much worse prognosis. The presence of a malignant squamous component, the adenosquamous carcinoma, appears to predict a similarly poor prognosis [23], although this may merely reflect the accompanying presence of a poorly differentiated glandular component [24]. In the GOG study, when stratified according to either depth of invasion or histologic grade, there was no statistically significant difference between adenocarcinoma and adenocarcinoma with squamous elements, with respect to the probability of pelvic or paraaortic lymph node metastasis or recurrence at three years. The GOG recommented that the terms adenoacanthoma and adenosquamous carcinoma be abandoned and replaced by 'adenocarcinoma with squamous differentiation,' since the prognosis of each category appeared to be the same [25].

Hendrikson et al. [26] have described a variant of endometrial carcinoma, papillary serous carcinoma, and have suggested a high incidence of deep myometrial invasion, a higher recurrence rate, and a propensity for intra-abdominal spread and recurrence.The group also had significantly reduced survival compared to standard endometrial carcinoma. These findings appear to have been confirmed by other reports of papillary carcinoma [27, 28]. A similarly poor prognosis appears to accompany clear-cell carcinoma of the endometrium. Forty-nine percent of Christopherson's 45 Stage I cases were dead at five years [29]. Webb reports only a 64% five-year survival rate among 29 cases compared to an 80% five-year survival for adenocarcinoma [30].

Less well-studied are the rarer forms, such as mucinous adenocarcinoma or pure squamous carcinomas. A recent review of 18 cases of mucinous adenocarcinoma suggests that the tumor is usually well differentiated and has a relatively good prognosis [31]. Care should be taken to avoid the diagnosis of adenosquamous carcinoma when normal endometrium contains squamous metaplasia, which may be misinterpreted on the specimen [32].

Histologic grade and myometrial invasion

A strong interrelationship between histologic grade, depth of myometrial invasion, lymph node metastasis, and prognosis has been repeatedly demonstrated in the literature and confirmed by the GOG data. Both histologic grade and myometrial invasion are independently and simultaneously related to the risk of lymph node metastasis (Table 3). Grade 3 lesions with deep myometrial invasion had the highest rate of nodal metastasis, with 34% showing positive pelvic nodes and 23% positive paraaortic nodes. The value of this information is that it is potentially available intraoperatively and it allows decisions regarding surgical management of individual patients to be made at the time of the surgery.

Adnexal and intraperitoneal spread

When endometrial carcinoma spreads beyond the uterus to the adnexae or more widely within the peritoneum, all series report a worse outcome, whether that spread be clinically apparent (and thus Stage III or IV), macroscopically detectable at surgery, or microscopic alone. The reported five-year survival for such groups are 16%, 40%, and 70% respectively [5]. The GOG data reports a 32% pelvic node and 20% aortic node metastasis rate associated with adnexal involvement and a 51% pelvic and 23% aortic metastasis rate with other extrauterine involvement [7]. Most significantly, if standard surgical and radiotherapeutic techniques are applied to this group of patients, a significant percentage will fail because their disease will, to a large but variable extent, be outside of standard treatment fields.

Cervical/isthmus involvement

Whether involvement of the cervix by endometrial cancer is clinically apparent or clinically occult (documented by endocervical curettage), the patient qualifies as Stage II, and most series report a decreased survival compared to Stage I. Most investigators report a worse survival for gross disease than for occult disease (Table 5), and the presence of histologically demonstrable stromal invasion on a hysterectomy specimen carries a worse prognosis than no invasion [44]. The latter series also showed that of patients with tumor fragments in the endocervical curettage specimen, 23% had cervical extension in the hysterectomy specimen, twice the rate of cases with a negative ECC. Not all series agree, however. The recent report from the M.D. Anderson Hospital showed a worse survival than for Stage I disease, but failed to demonstrate a survival difference between gross cervical involvement, occult stromal involvement and these with no evidence of stromal invasion [34]. They reported five-year survivals of 70%, 64%, and 65% respectively, figures that are better across-the-board than many other figures for this stage of disease.

Of further interest is the relationship of histologic grade and myometrial invasion to outcome in Stage II endometrial cancer. In the predominately surgical series of Homesley et al. [35], a major survival relationship to myometrial invasion (68% with <1/3 versus 48% with >1/3) was observed. Grigsby et al. report a significant decrease in survival with Grade 3 disease when compared to Grades 1 and 2 (75% versus 50%, ten-year survival) [41].

These data point out the shortcomings of the clinical diagnosis of occult State II endometrial carcinoma and raise questions about the significance of cervical involvement as a risk factor independent of histologic grade and myometrial invasion, especially in the absence of cervical stromal invasion. Consequently, we approach occult Stage II disease as if it were Stage I (see below).

Peritoneal cytology, vascular space invasion, and hormone receptors

These final factors are of clear importance (Table 5). Since this information is not usually available at the time of surgery, even though each may

Table 5. Frequency of nodal metastasis among risk factors.

Risk factors		Pelvic		Aortic	
		No. (%)	Significance (p-value)	No. (%)	Significance (p-value)
Stage					
Ia	(N=346)	23 (7%)	0.01	11 (3%)	0.008
Ib	(N=275)	35 (13%)			
Grade					
1 Well	(N=180)	5 (3%)	<0.0001	3 (2%)	<0.0007
2 Moderate	(N=288)	25 (9%)		14 (5%)	
3 Poor	(N=153)	28 (18%)		7 (11%)	
Myometrial invasion					
Endometrial only	(N=87)	1 (1%)	<0.0001	1 (1%)	<0.0001
Superficial	(N=279)	15 (5%)		8 (3%)	
Middle	(N=116)	7 (6%)		1 (1%)	
Deep	(N=139)	35 (25%)		24 (17%)	
Peritoneal cytology					
Negative	(N=537)	38 (7%)	<0.0001	20 (4%)	<0.0001
Positive	(N=75)	19 (25%)		14 (19%)	
Site of tumor location					
Fundus	(N=524)	42 (8%)	0.01	20 (4%)	0.0001
Isthmus-cervix	(N=97)	16 (16%)		14 (14%)	
Adenexal involvement					
Positive	(N=34)	11 (32%)	0.0001	7 (20%)	0.0003
Negative	(N=587)	47 (8%)		27 (5%)	
Other extrauterine metastasis					
Positive	(N=35)	18 (51%)	0.0001	8 (23%)	0.0001
Negative	(N=586)	40 (7%)		26 (4%)	
Capillary-like space involvement					
Positive	(N=93)	21 (27%)	0.0001	15 (19%)	0.0001
Nagative	(N=528)	37 (7%)		19 (9%)	

Adapted from Creasman et al. [7].

significantly alter the final prognosis and treatment plan, they need not be considered in planning the surgical approach.

Surgery for Stage I endometrial carcinoma

The ability to obtain such detailed prognostic information at the time of laparotomy has lead to the current trend towards surgery as the primary treatment for endometrial carcinoma. Furthermore, failure to document that routine preoperative radiation therapy improves the survival of patients with this disease [42, 43, 44] indicates that a laparotomy, total abdominal hysterectomy and bilateral salpingo-oophorectomy, peritoneal cytology, and individualized surgical staging should be the mainstay of treatment for those patients with Stage I or occult Stage II disease (Figure 2).

Selecting the incision

Although the midline suprapublic incision is traditionally recommended when operating for genital cancer, providing good exposure and allowing extension superiorly if necessary, the low transverse incision is commonly employed in gynecologic surgery. In endometrial cancer the probability that a low transverse incision will be inadequate is substantial, especially in the presence of a moderately-to-poorly differentiated malignancy, an enlarged uterus, cervical extension, or an adnexal tumor. In these situations, omentectomy and removal or biopsy of enlarged aortic nodes and abdominal metastases may be necessary. The low transverse incision does not usually permit these procedures. Sometimes the abdominal contents cannot even be adequately explored, let alone safely operated on, using a low transverse incision. An inadequate vertical incision, of course, is similarly limiting.

Exploration

After the abdominal incision is complete and the peritoneal cavity is opened, a note is made of any ascites present. If any are present, the fluid is collected for cytologic examination. If not, sterile, warm saline is introduced into the pelvis and used to bathe the anterior pouch and posterior cul-de-sac. It is then withdrawn, placed into a sterile bottle, and transferred to the cytologic laboratory for further processing. Additional specimens for cytology can be taken from the paracolic gutters and over the liver, according to the established practice in ovarian cancer. Next, a systematic exploration of the abdominal contents is carried out with special concern for the liver, retroperitoneal nodes, and omentum.

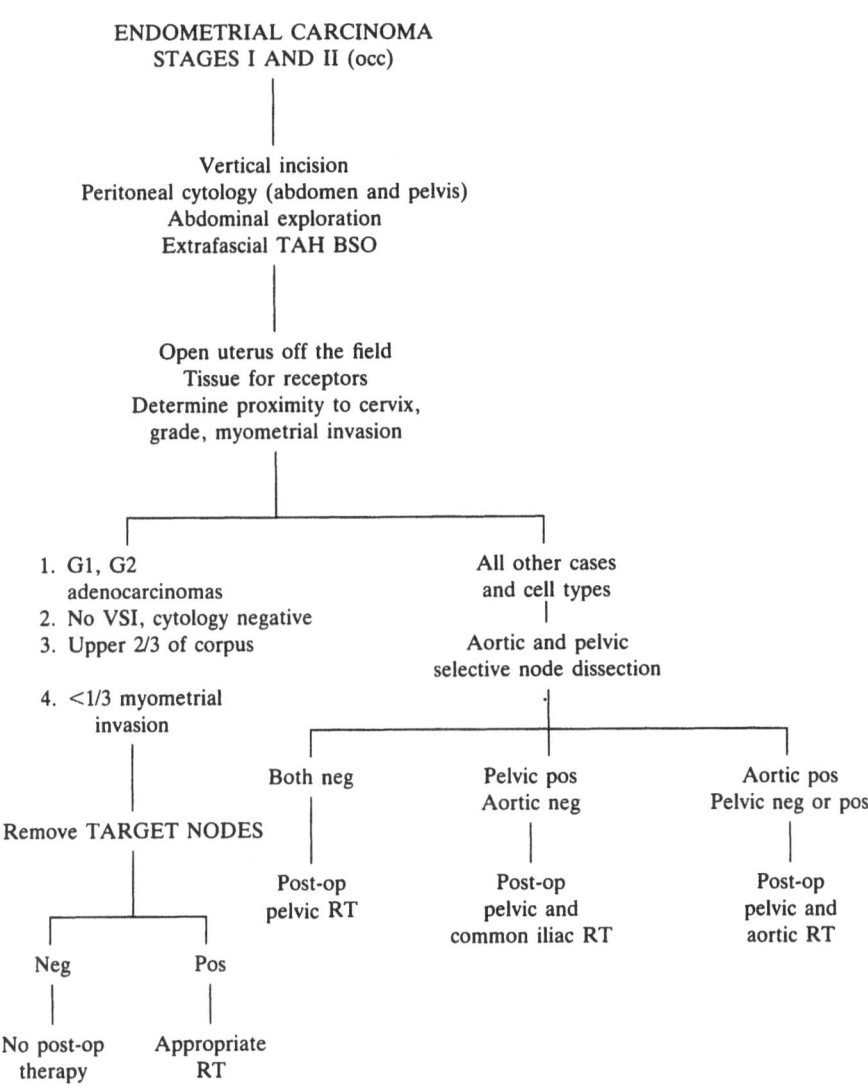

ENDOMETRIAL CARCINOMA
STAGES I AND II (occ)

Vertical incision
Peritoneal cytology (abdomen and pelvis)
Abdominal exploration
Extrafascial TAH BSO

Open uterus off the field
Tissue for receptors
Determine proximity to cervix,
grade, myometrial invasion

1. G1, G2
   adenocarcinomas
2. No VSI, cytology negative
3. Upper 2/3 of corpus

4. <1/3 myometrial
   invasion

All other cases
and cell types

Aortic and pelvic
selective node dissection

Remove TARGET NODES

Both neg

Pelvic pos
Aortic neg

Aortic pos
Pelvic neg or pos

Neg   Pos

Post-op
pelvic RT

Post-op
pelvic and
common iliac RT

Post-op
pelvic and
aortic RT

No post-op   Appropriate
therapy   RT

Figure 2. Protocol for management of clinical Stage I and II (occult) encometrial carcinoma. Total abdominal hysterectomy. bilateral salpingo-oophorectomy. Target nodes are removed for frozen section analysis first. If they are positive, a blind, selective node dissection in that areas is unnecessary. If there are multiple or large aortic node metastases, the scalene fat pad should be removed. Metastasis at that level would be a contraindication to extended field radiation therapy. RT = radiation therapy, Pos = metastases present, VSI = vascular space invasion, Neg = metastases absent.

Adapted from Morrow and Townsend [48].

Abdominal hysterectomy

The hysterectomy is begun by placing a Pean clamp across the upper broad ligament on each side of the uterus, excompassing the tube, the utero-ovarian ligament, and the round ligament. The Pean clamps are used to manipulate the uterus without compressing it. Uterine elevators, tenacula, and myometrial traction should not be employed, to avoid the possible risk of intravascular dissemination from traumatizing the cancer-containing uterus.

After dividing the round ligaments, the anterior broad ligament peritoneum is incised across the vesico-uterine reflection. Posteriorly, the peritioneal incision is extended lateral and parallel to the ovarian vessels in the infundibulopelvic ligament. By gentle traction on the uterus and broad ligament, the lateral peritoneum is separated from the pelvic wall, exposing the ureter, iliac vessels, and obturator fossa. Any enlarged or suspicious nodes are removed for histologic examination. With the ureter under direct vision, the ovarian vessels are divided well proximal to the ovary. After developing the vesicovaginal space to a level below the cervix, the uterine vessels are skeletonized and divided at the isthmus. The major vascular drainage of the uterus has now been ligated with minimal uterine manipulation. The cardinal ligaments are incised down to the level of the lateral vaginal fornices, the vagina is divided at its interface with the cervix, and the uterus is delivered from the pelvis. No attempt is made to specifically remove a cuff of vagina. The vaginal cuff is closed, and the pelvis is irrigated with saline.

The uterus is then opened off the field, and the status of the tumor is evaluated, particularly with regard to the major prognostic features that dictate if extended surgical staging is indictated. Frozen section may be necessary. When there is sufficient tissue, estrogen and progesterone receptor content of the cancer should be determined, ensuring that the specimen submitted for receptor analysis is, in fact, malignant tissue. Frozen section documentation is recommended [45]. Clinically obvious metastases should be biopsied and analyzed separately, as they may have different receptor status from the primary tumor [46].

A rational decision regarding assessment of pelvic, common iliac, or aortic nodes can be made intraoperatively on the basis of the intraoperative pathology examination of the specimen. The GOG data has provided a multivariant analysis restricted to those factors that were predictive of lymph node metastasis and that are known preoperatively or intraoperatively. Using the grade of tumor and the depth of invasion, the incidence of lymph node metastasis can be estimated (Table 6), and the risk for each patient can be defined as low, moderate, or high. The clinician can then decide whether or not to perform a lymphadenectomy. Enlarged or suspicious nodes should be removed, regardless of presumed risk of nodal metastasis.

Excluding patients with obvious extrauterine metastasis, there were no

Table 6. Determination of risk factors for nodal metatasis using multivariant analysis.

Risk factor	Lymph node metastasis	
	Pelvic	Aortic
Low risk		
(No moderate or high risk factors)		
Grade 1. endometrium only. no intraperitoneal disease	0/44 (0%)	0/44 (0%)
Moderate risk		
(Inner mid invasion, Grade 2–3 — no intraperitoneal		
disease)	4/158 (3%)	3/158 (2%)
Only one factor	15/268 (6%)	6/268 (2%)
Both factors		
High Risk		
(Intraperitoneal disease, deep myometrial invasion)	21/116 (18%)	17/116 (15%)
Deep invasion only	4/12 (33%)	1/12 (8%)
Intraperitoneal disease only	14/23 (61%)	7/23 (30%)
Both		

Adapted from Creasman et al. [7].

patients with well-differentiated lesions and no myometrial invasion in the GOG study with positive nodes. Therefore, lymphadenectomy is not indicated as a routine in these patients. Conversely, patients with high-risk factors have a high enough rate of lymph node metastasis to warrant pelvic lymphadenectomies. Regarding the aortic nodes, all categories are at low risk except the Grade 2 and 3, outer one-third group, which are at high risk. Two groups, however, had too few patients to make confident predictions: the Grade 3, no invasion (zero of nine pelvic or aortic metastasis), and Grade 1, outer one-third (one of 16 had both pelvic and aortic node metastasis).

In the moderate-risk category, if Grade 2 tumors, Grade 3 tumors, or inner or mid-myometrial invasion was present, four of 158 (3%) had pelvic metastasis. When both factors applied, that is either Grade 2 or 3 with (superficial or middle) myometrial invasion, then 15 of 268 patients (6%) had positive pelvic nodes. The risk when both factors is present, particularly for large tumors, probably justifies pelvic and aortic lymph node dissection.

Of particular note is that the surgeon should not determine whether lymphadenectomy is done on the basis of palpation of the nodal area alone. In the GOG study, less than 10% of patients with metastasis to lymph nodes had grossly enlarged nodes [7].

When high risk features exist in the absence of target nodes, the lower aortic nodes can be exposed by incising the peritoneum over the lower aorta and the right common iliac artery. Mobilizing the cecum and terminal ileum gives better exposure of the caval region. After identifying the ureter and ovarian vessels laterally, the aorta and the common iliac artery medially, and the duodenum or base of the inferior mesenteric artery superiorly, the fat pad overlying the vena cava within this anatomic area is removed. The peritoneal incision is then closed.

Wound closure

For the vertical midline incision, we recommend the Smead–Jones closure with either continuous or interrupted monofilament No. 1–2 guage nylon or Prolene suture. If the patient is thin, the knots can be buried or the longer lasting absorbable sutures, such as polydioxanone (PDS), can be used, depending on the risk for wound disruption. No sutures are placed in the subcutaneous tissue, but if the patient is obese, a closed vacuum drainage system is inserted. The would is irrigated with saline before the skin is closed. In the very obese patient, interrupted subcuticular Dexon or Vicryl sutures give added support to the skin.

Surgery for Stage II endometrial carcinoma

Bearing in mind the above discussion regarding the prognostic significance of cervical involvement, our approach to the patient with occult Stage II disease differs little from the patient with clinical Stage I. The major difference is that since even surface endocervical involvement appears to carry a worse prognosis, all of these patients should have pelvic and paraaortic lymph node dissection.

When the cervix is clinically involved by adenocarcinoma and the endometrium also contains cancerous tissue, we treat the patient the same as if she had cervical carcinoma, i.e., by radical hysterectomy with pelvic and paraaortic lymphadenectomy, if the cervical lesion is less than 4 cm in diameter, or by pelvic and intracavitary irradiation followed by adjuvant simple hysterectomy for larger lesions. In the former case, if the pelvic and aortic nodes, the surgical margins, and the washings are negative, no further adjuvant therapy is needed. The decision to perform radical hysterectomy is not a common one, taking into account the average age of these patients and the high incidence of associated medical problems, such as obesity, cardiovascular disease, and diabetes.

Surgery for Stage III and IV endometrial carcinoma

Patients presenting with clinical Stage III or IV disease are an assorted group, and surgical therapy needs to be highly individualized according to the specific details for each patient. A number of points can be made in general, however. First, accurate surgical staging is important even in the presence of presumed extrauterine extension. In the series of 62 patients from Toronto with Stage III disease, 13 patients underwent laparotomy: eight were confirmed surgical Stage III, but five were downstaged and one was upstaged [47]. Patients placed in the Stage III category on the basis of an adnexal mass should undergo surgery without preoperative radiation therapy, to determine the nature of the mass (inflammatory, synchronous ovarian primary cancer, metastasis), to perform hysterectomy, and to perform tumor reductive surgery.

Surgically resectable disease, even when advanced, has a much better prognosis than its unresectable counterpart. Aalders et al. reported the same five-year survival for completely resected Stage III cases (40%) as for microscopic or subclinical extrauterine tumor [5]. This compared with an 11% five-year survival for patients with incomplete resection. But in only 14 of 108 cases (13%) could such optimal surgery be performed. These findings appear to be confirmed by Mackillop's series, in which patients with no residual disease after surgery had a 79.5% five-year survival compared to 23% when disease remained [42]. Although the accumulated data is smaller, it would appear that advanced endometrial cancer behaves like ovarian cancer, and the goals of surgical diagnosis and resection are probably equivalent. When adjuvant chemotherapy is used in this setting, a 'second look' laparotomy at the completion of chemotherapy, based on the ovarian model, is probably warranted.

Patients who have Stage III endometrial carcinoma by virtue of vaginal or parametrial extension are given pelvic radiation therapy after a thorough metastatic survey. When the therapy is complete, exploratory laparotomy is recommended to document disease extension beyond the treatment field. The choice between extended field radiation therapy, chemotherapy, or hormone therapy can then be made on the rational knowledge of true disease extent. Hysterectomy can be accomplished at this time if the parameteria are clear. Laparoscopy prior to radiotherapy may be useful for selected cases to rule out intraperitoneal disease.

Conclusion

Enough is known about endometrial carcinoma, particularly in early stage, to confidently predict the risk of extrauterine metastasis, recurrence, and survival. This information is best obtained by using a primary surgical approach to these patients and individualizing the surgery for each patient, based on the presence or absence of well-established prognostic factors. Apart from being the mainstay of treatment, such an approach will identify those patients requiring adjuvant therapy (and, importantly, those who don't) and help determine that such adjuvant therapy is adequate and appropriate for the true extent of the disease. Such an approach will, it is hoped, lead to a rational use of therapy and minimize both undertreatment and overtreatment.

References

1. Cancer Facts and Figures — 1987. New York: American Cancer Society.
2. Keller D, Kempson RL, Levine G, McLennon C, 1974. Management of the Patient with Early Endometrial Carcinoma. Cancer 33:1108.
3. Malkasian GD, 1978. Carcinoma of the Endometrium: Effect of Stage and Grade on Survival. Cancer 41:996.
4. FIGO, 1985. Annual Report on Gynecologigal Cancer. International Federation of Gynecology and Obstetrics, Vol 19.
5. Aalders JG, Abeler V, Kolstad P, 1984. Clinical (Stage 3) as compared to subclinical intrapelvic tumor spread in endometrial carcinoma: A clinical and histopathological study of 175 patients. Gynecol Oncol 17:64.
6. Chambers SK, Kapp DS, Peschel RE, et al., 1987. Prognostic Factors and Sites of Failure in FIGO Stage I, Grade 3 Endometrial Carcinoma.
7. Creasman WT, Morrow CP, Bundy BN, et al., 1987. Surgical Pathologic Spread Patterns of Endometrial Carcinoma. A Gynecologic Oncology Group Study. Cancer 60:2035–2041.
8. FIGO 1973. Annual Report on Gynecological Cancer. International Federation of Gynecology and Obstetrics, Vol 15.
9. Wharton JT, Mikuta JJ, Mettlin C, 1986. Risk Factors in the Current Management in Carcinoma of the Endometrium. Surg Gynecol Obstet 162:515–520.
10. Schink JC, Lurain JR, Wallemark CB, Chmiel JS, 1987. Tumor Size in Endometrial Cancer: A Prognostic Factor for Lymph Node Metastasis. Obstet Gynecol 70:216–219.
11. Hricak, Stern JL, Fisher MR, et al., 1987. Endometrial Carcinoma Staging by MR Imaging. Radiology 162:297–305.
12. Mettler FA, Christie JH, Garcia JF, et al. 1981. Radionuclide Liver and Bone Scanning in the Evaluation of Patients with Endometrial Carcinoma. Radiology 141:777–780.
13. Nori D, Hilaris BS, Tome M, et al. 1987. Combined Surgery and Radiation in Endometrial Carcinoma: An Analysis of Prognostic Factors. Int J Radiation Oncology Biol Physics 13:489–497.
14. Duk JM, Aalders JG, Fleuren GJ, de Bruijn HWA, 1986. CA–125: A useful Marker in Endometrial Carcinoma. Am J Obstet Gynecol 155:1097–1102.
15. Patsner B, Mann WJ, Cohen H, Loesch M, 1988. Predictive Value of Pre-operative Serum CA–125 Levels in Clinically Localized and Advanced Endometrial Carcinoma. Presented at 19th Annual Meeting, Society of Gynecologic Oncologists, Miami, February, 1988.
16. Frick HC, Munnell EW, Richart RM, et al., 1973. Carcinoma of the Endometrium. Am J Obstet Gynecol 115:663.
17. De Palo G, Kenda R, Andreola S, Luciano L. Musumeci R, Rilke F, 1982. Endometrial Carcinoma Stage I. Obstet Gynecol 60:225–231.
18. Kauppila A, Kojansuu E, Vihko R, 1982. Cytosol estrogen and progestin receptors in endometrial carcinoma patients treated with surgery, radioterapy, and progestin. Cancer 50:2157.
19. Aalders JG, Abeler V, Kolstad P, 1980. Postoperative external irradiation and prognostic parameters in Stage I endometrial carcinoma. Obstet Gynecol 56:419.
20. Lotocki RJ, Copeland LJ, DePetrillo AD, Muirhead W, 1983. Stage I endometrial carcinoma: Treatment results in 835 patients. Am J Obstet Gynecol 146:141–145.
21. Bokham JV, 1981. Two Pathogenetic Types of Endometrial Carcioma. Gynecol Oncol 15:10–17.
22. Quinn MA, Kneale BJ, and Fortune DW, 1985. Endometrial Carcinoma in Premenopausal Women: A Clinicopathological Study. Gynecol Oncol 20:298–306.
23. Christopherson WM, Connelly PJ, Alberhasky RC, 1983. Carcinoma of the Endometrium. V. An analysis of prognosticators in patients with favorable subtypes and Stage I disease. Cancer 51:1705.
24. Silverberg SG, Bolin MG, DeGiorgi LS, 1972. Adenocanthoma and mixed adeono-

quamous carcinoma of the endometrium: A clinicopathologic study. Cancer 30:1307–1314.

25. Zaino RJ, Kurman R, Herbold D, et al., 1988. The significance of squamous differentiation in endometrial carcinoma. Presented at 19th Annual Meeting of the Society of Gynecologic Oncologists, Miami, February, 1988.

26. Hendrikson M, Ross J, Eifel PJ, et al., 1982. Adenocarcinoma of the endometrium: Analysis of 256 cases with carcinoma limited to the endometrium. Gynecol Oncol 13:373.

27. Christopherson WM, Alberhasky RC, Connelly PJ, 1982. Carcinoma of the endometrium II: Papillary adenocarcinoma: A clinical pathological study of 46 cases. Am J Clin Path 77:534.

28. Ramirez–Gonzalez CE, Adamsons K, Mangual–Vasquez TY, Wallach RC, 1987. Papillary adenocarcinoma in the endometrium. Obstet Gynecol 70:212–215.

29. Christopherson WM, Alberhasky RC, Connelly PJ, 1982. Carcinoma of the endometrium: I. A clinicopathological study of clear-cell carcinoma and secretory carcinoma. Cancer 49:1511.

30. Webb GA, Lagios MD, 1986. Clear cell carcinoma of the endometrium. Am J Obstet Gynecol 156:1486–1491.

31. Melham MF, Tobon H, 1987. Mucinous adenocarcinoma of the endometrium: A clinico-pathological review of 18 cases. Int J Gynecol Path 6:347–355.

32. Anderson WA, Taylor PT, Fechner RE, Pinkerton JV, 1987. Endometrial metaplasia associated with endometrial adenocarcinoma. Am J Obstet Gynecol 157:597–604.

33. Morrow CP. Prognostic factors in endometrial cancer. Annual Clinical Conference on Cancer, Vol 29. Gynecol. Cancer: Diagnosis and treatment strategies. University of Texas System Cancer Center.

34. Larson DM, Copeland LJ, Gallagher HS, Gershenson DM, Freedman RS, Wharton JT, Kline RC, 1987. Nature of cervical involvement in endometrial carcinoma. Cancer 59:959–962.

35. Kinsella TJ, Bloomer WD, Lavin PT, Knapp RC, 1980. Stage II Endometrial Carcinoma: 10 year follow up of combined radiation and surgical treatment. Gynecol Oncol 10:290.

36. Homesley HD, Boronow RC, Lewis JL, 1977. Stage II endometrial adenocarcinoma: Memorial Hospital for cancer, 1949–1965. Obstet Gynecol 49:604.

37. Onsrud M, Aalders J, Abeler V, Taylor P, 1982. Endometrial Carcinoma with Cervical involvement (Stage II): Prognostic factors and value of combined radiological-surgical treatment. Gynecol Oncol 13:76.

38. Bruckman JE, Bloomer WD, Marck A, Ehrmann RI, Knapp RC, 1980. Stage III adenocarcinoma of endometrium: Two prognostic groups. Gynecol Oncol 9:12.

39. Boronow RC, 1973. A fresh look corpus cancer management. Obstet Gynecol 42:448–451.

40. Bigelow B, Vekstein V, Demopoulos RI, 1983. Endometrial carcinoma Stage II: Route and extent of spread to the cervix. Obstet Gynecol 62:363.

41. Grigsby PW, Kuske RR, Perez CA, et al., 1987. Medically inoperable Stage I adenocarcinoma of the endometrium treated with radiotherapy alone. Int J Radiation Oncol Biol Physics 13:483–488.

42. Aalders J, Abeler V, Kolstad P, Onsrud M, 1980. Postoperative external irradiation and prognostic parameters in Stage I endometrial carcinoma. Obstete Gynecol 56:419–427.

43. Piver MS, Yazigi R, Blumenson L, Tsukada Y, 1979. A prospective trial comparing hysterectomy, hysterectomy plus vaginal readium, and uterine radium plus hysterectomy in Stage I endometrial carcinoma. Obstet Gynecol 54:85–89.

44. Fanning J, Evans MC, Peters AJ, et al., 1987. Adjuvant radiotherapy for Stage I, Grade 2 endometrial adenocarcinoma and adenocanthoma with limited myometrial invasion. Obstet Gynecol 70:920–922.

45. Quinn MA, Cauchi M, Fortune D, 1985. Endometrial carcinoma: steroid receptors and response to medroxy progesterone acetate. Gynecol Oncol 21:314.

46. Utaaker E, Iverson OE, Skaarland E, 1987. The distribution and prognostic implications of steroid receptors in endometrial carcinomas. Gynec Oncol 28:89–100.

47. Mackillop WJ, Pringle JF. Stage III endometrial carcinoma. A review of 90 cases. Cancer 56:2519.
48. Morrow CP, Townsend DE, 1987. Synopsis of Gynecologic Oncology, 3rd Edition. New York: Wiley.

3. Peritoneal cytology in endometrial carcinoma

Gregory P. Sutton

Introduction

Although interest in the cytologic composition of peritoneal fluid in gynecologic and other malignancies is evident in publications dating to the turn of
the century [1], the clinical importance of malignant cells present in ascites
or peritoneal washings was not addressed until 1956, when Keettel and
Elkins [2] reported their preliminary experience with peritoneal cytology in
ovarian cancer. In 1961, Morton et al. [3] demonstrated malignant cells in
peritoneal fluid in the majority of patients with advanced ovarian carcinoma
and suggested that the absence of malignant cells in early ovarian cancer
might indicate a favorable prognosis.

Malkasian et al. [4] reported a five-year survival of 90% in patients with
Stage Ia$_1$ Grade 1 ovarian epithelial tumors and contrasted this to five-year
survivals of 68% and 56% for patients with Stage I lesions featuring excresc-
ences or tumor rupture. The reduced survival was attributed to microscopic
seeding of the peritoneal cavity with malignant cells from the primary
tumor. Keettel et al. [5] subsequently reported positive cytology in 16 of
44 patients with carcinoma clinically confined to one or both ovaries and
suggested that treatment of these patients with intraperitoneal radioactive
gold could improve five-year survival from 63.3% to 92.8%.

In 1975, the International Federation of Gynecology and Obstetrics
(FIGO) adopted the use of the 'C' subclassification in Stage I and II ovarian
carcinoma to designate the presence of ascites or malignant peritoneal
cytology, underwriting the concept that the presence of either implied a
worse prognosis than for comparable patients without these features.

In endometrial adenocarcinoma, the significance of malignant peritoneal
cytology has been much less well defined than in ovarian cancer. In 1958,
Keettel and Pixley [6] reported three cases of malignant cytology in endometrial cancer and later [5] updated this to five of 39 (12%) patients with
Stage I endometrial adenocarcinoma, two of whom had experienced uterine
perforation at the time of curettage prior to hysterectomy. Morton et al. [3]
reported four cases of patients with positive cytology among 24 endometrial
carcinomas (16.7%) and suggested that the source of these malignant cells

E. Surwit and D. Alberts (eds.), ENDOMETRIAL CANCER. Copyright © 1989.
Kluwer Academic Publishers, Boston. All rights reserved.

might be transtubal passage from the endometrium into the peritoneal cavity.

In 1962, Marcus [7] presented three patients with malignant peritoneal cytology and no evidence of extrauterine spread at the time of surgery, two of whom succumbed to recurrent disease shortly after initial operation. He suggested that the finding of malignant cytology in endometrial cancer was a grave prognostic indicator.

In 1971, Creasman and Rutledge [8] summarized the experience with peritoneal cytology at M.D. Anderson Hospital and found malignant peritoneal cytology in 11.5% (21/183) of patients with endometrial cancer of all stages undergoing exploratory surgery. All had received preoperative radiation therapy and only 63% had persistent disease in the uterus at the time of surgery. A threefold increase in the risk of positive washings with myometrial invasion was noted in this review, and absolute four-year survival for all stages was poorer in those patients with positive cytology (p = 0.003).

Ten years later, Creasman et al. [9] reported findings from a Gynecologic Oncology Group pilot study from Duke University, the University of Mississippi, and the University of Southern California. In this study, 26 of 167 (15.5%) patients with Stage I disease, many of whom had received preoperative radiation therapy, were found to have positive washings. Thirteen of these patients had extrauterine disease at laparotomy. Six of the 13 lacking extrauterine spread died of intraperitoneal carcinomatosis, suggesting a relationship between malignant cytology and subsequent intraperitoneal recurrence.

Studies such as that of Yazigi et al. [10] claimed that the finding of positive cytology had no clinical impact. In their study, recurrence rates and actuarial five-year and ten-year survival statistics were unaffected by the presence of positive peritoneal washings. In their study there is a relatively small number of patients, and 30% of those with positive washings were lost to intercurrent disease.

Konski et al. [11] reached similar conclusions in a retrospective review of 134 Stage I patients with endometrial cancer. No survival differences were noted in this study. Survival comparisons between patients with benign and malignant peritoneal washings are obscured by the fact that all those with malignant cytology received either pelvic or abdominal radiotherapy.

Indiana University–St. Vincent Hospital study

To further determine the role of peritoneal cytology in endometrial cancer, records of 615 patients from 1971 to 1986 at Indiana University Medical Center and St. Vincent Hospital, Indianapolis, were reviewed [12]. Peritoneal washings were obtained for cytologic examination in 340 patients; these patients comprised the study group. Seventy-five (27.2%) patients with clinical Stage I disease received preoperative pelvic radiotherapy with or without an implant. Fifty-seven (20.7%) patients with clinical Stage I disease received postoperative pelvic or extended field radiotherapy. All patients with Stages II and III disease received radiotherapy, and patients with Stage IV disease were treated with adjunctive hormonal therapy, radiotherapy, or chemotherapy when appropriate. In 40% of patients with clinical Stage I disease and positive peritoneal cytology, adjunctive hormonal therapy with oral megestrol or medroxyprogesterone acetate was given postoperatively.

Peritoneal washings were obtained at the time of initial exploration in all patients by instilling 100 ml of sterile balanced salt solution over the pelvic viscera after the small bowel had been manually elevated. The solution was aspirated from the posterior cul-de-sac and sent directly to the cytology laboratory, where volume was measured before the sample was divided into two centrifuge tubes and spun down. The precipitate was smeared directly onto slides and fixed in 95% ethyl alcohol before being stained by a modified Papanicolaou technique. When only a very small amount of precipitate was obtained, slides were prepared using the Shandon Cytospin 2 (Shandon Southern Instruments, Inc.) before fixation and staining. Any remaining precipitate was processed into formalin-fixed cell blocks from which slides were cut. Criteria for establishing the presence of malignant cells were those described by Koss [13].

For the 340 patients, 75 peritoneal specimens were reported to contain malignant cells. Three cases (4.0%) were considered false positives upon cytologic review and were excluded, leaving 72 true positive specimens, or 21.3% of the series. No false negatives were identified. Forty-seven (17.1%) patients with clinical Stage I disease, eight (19.5%) with clinical Stage II disease, and 17 (68.7%) patients with clinical Stage III disease were found to have positive washings, a significant stage-related trend (P < 0.001, chi square test, Table 1). When patients with clinical Stage I were divided by substage, 14 of 127, or 11.0%, of those with Stage IA and 27 of 121, or 22.3%, of those with Stage IB had malignant cytology. This difference was also statistically significant (P = 0.03, chi square test).

In clinical Stage I disease, increasing histologic grade was associated with an increasing risk of positive cytology. Of 104 Grade 1 and 103 Grade 2 tumors, ten (9.6%) and 18 (17.5%), respectively, had positive washings. In

Table 1. Peritoneal cytology and clinical stage.

Stage	N	Malignant	% Malignant
I	276	47	17.1
II	41	8	19.5
III	16	11	68.7
IV	7	6	85.7
Total	340	72	21.2

P < 0.001, chi square test.

43

Table 2. Clinical Stage I: Histologic grade and malignant cytology.

Grade	N	Malignant	% Malignant
1	104	10	9.6
2	103	18	17.5
3	41	13	31.7

P = 0.002, chi square test.

Table 3. Clinical Stage I: Myometrial invasion and malignant cytology.

Invasion	N	Malignant	% Malignant
None or inner third	185	24	13.0
Middle third	28	5	17.9
Outer third	35	12	34.9

P = 0.003, chi square test.

contrast, 13 of 41 (31.7%) of patients with Grade 3 tumors had positive cytology (p = 0.002, chi square test for trend, Table 2). A similar relationship was found between the depth of myometrial invasion and positive peritoneal cytology. Malignant washings were identified in 24 of 185 (13.0%) patients with myometrial invasion limited to the inner third, in five of 28 (17.9%) patients with middle-third invasion, and in 12 of 35 (34.9%) patients with outer third invasion (Table 3). This trend also achieves statistical significance (P = 0.003, chi square test for trend).

In patients with clinical Stage I endometrial cancer, those with adnexal metastases were significantly more likely to have malignant peritoneal cytology than those patients without extrauterine spread. Of seventeen patients with adnexal spread, eight, or 47.1%, were found to have malignant peritoneal washings compared to 33 of 231 (14.3%) of those with negative adnexae (P < 0.001, chi square test).

Seventy-eight patients with clinical Stage I disease had pelvic and para-aortic lymph node sampling prior to radiotherapy. Three of four patients (75%) with positive pelvic nodes and four of five patients (80%) with positive para-aortic nodes had malignant cytology. An association between node metastases and malignant cytology is suggested.

Patients with clinical Stage I disease in whom surgical findings indicated a higher surgical stage were more likely to have positive peritoneal cytology than those patients with surgical Stage I disease. Six of eleven (54.5%) patients with surgical Stages II-IV had malignant cytology, whereas nine of 67 (13.4%) patients with surgical Stage I disease had positive washings (P = 0.005, Fisher's Exact Test).

When all stages are examined and deaths from other causes are eliminated, 252 of 268 patients (94.0%) with benign peritoneal cytology survived disease-free, versus 38 of 72 patients (52.8%) with malignant cytology (P <

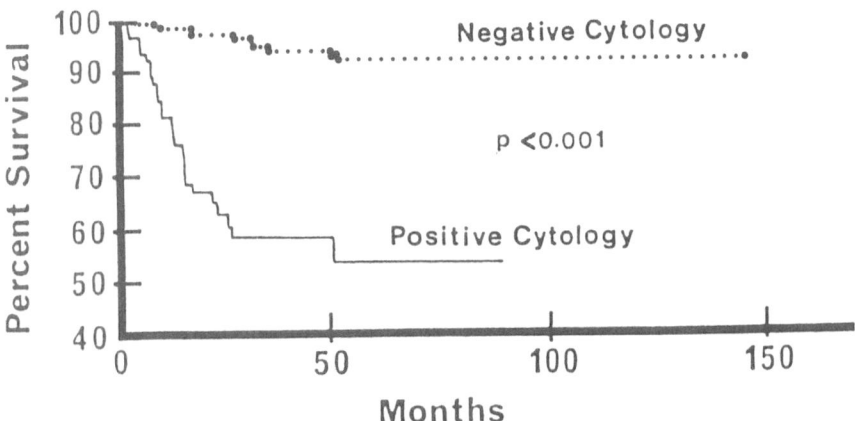

Figure 1. Survival in all patients by cytologic findings.

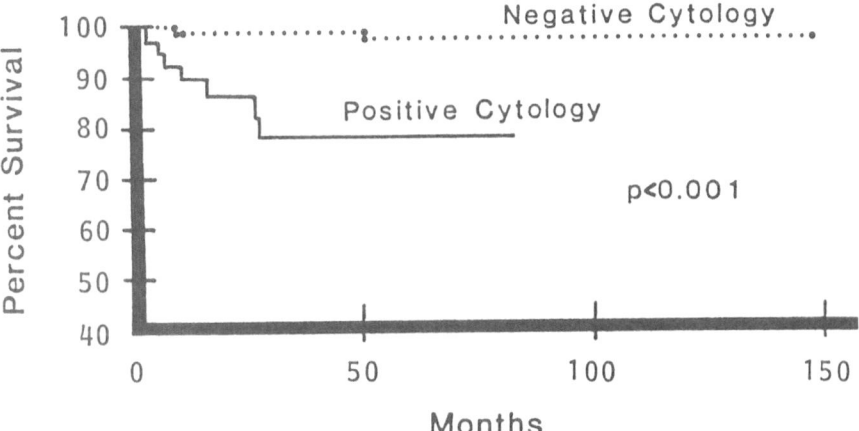

Figure 2. Survival in clinical Stage I by cytologic findings.

0.001). Survival for all stages was also significantly better for patients with benign cytology (Figure 1, P < 0.001).

In patients with clinical Stage I disease, 201 of 207 (97.1%) with negative cytology are disease-free survivors, versus 29 of 41 (70.7%) with positive washings (P < 0.001). Survival of patients with clinical Stage I disease and negative peritoneal cytology (204/207, 98.6%) is also superior when compared with those with malignant cytology (34 of 41, 82.9%) (Figure 2, P < 0.001). The use of progestational agents did not influence survival; radio-active isotopes were not employed in this study.

Complete surgical staging, including abdominal hysterectomy, bilateral salpingo-oophorectomy, and pelvic and para-aortic lymph node biopsies, was performed in 78 patients. Seventy-three of these patients had surgical

45

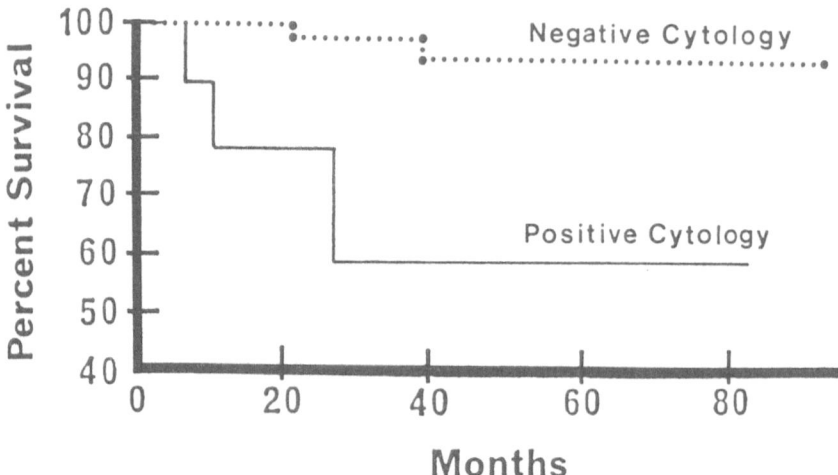

Figure 3. Disease-free survival in surgical Stage I by Cytologic findings.

Stage I tumors. Of the 11 patients in this group with positive cytology, three have died of cancer and eight (72.7%) survive without disease. Among the 62 patients with benign cytology, there have been two recurrences and no deaths. Disease-free survival is better in the latter group, although the small populations do not allow proper application of survival analysis (Figure 3).

A Cox proportional hazards regression model was utilized to determine the relative contributions of clinical stage, histologic grade, age, results of peritoneal cytology, depth of myometrial penetration, and presence or absence of adnexal metastases to survival among those patients where peritoneal cytology was available. After modeling, depth of myometrial invasion and the presence or absence of adnexal metastases did not correlate with survival. Clinical stage, histologic grade, age, and the results of peritoneal cytology are correlated with survival in this model, with the strengths of correlation expressed by increasing chi-square values in Table 4.

Of the twelve patients with clinical Stage I disease and malignant cytology who developed recurrences, nine (75%) had an intra-abdominal component. In contrast, of the six patients with clinical Stage I disease and benign cytology who developed recurrent disease, only one (16.7%) was intra-abdominal (Table 5).

Review

The incidence of malignant peritoneal cytology reported in nine discrete studies is presented in Table 6. The incidence of positive washings in Stage I disease approximates 14% from these studies, although differences in preoperative therapy exist. The Gynecologic Oncology Group series [14]

Table 4. Cox proportional hazards analysis of clinical variables.

Variable	X^2	P-value	R
Clinical stage	14.18	.0002	.220
Grade	10.99	.0009	.185
Age	7.87	.005	.153
Peritoneal cytology	4.66	.031	.103
Myometrial depth	1.96	.161	
Adnexal metastasis	0.00	.963.	

Table 5. Recurrences in clinical Stage I endometrial carcinoma by peritoneal cytology.

Site	Months
Malignant Cytology	
Abdomen	3.5
Abdomen	11.0
Abdomen	13.0
Abdomen	22.0
Abdomen	26.0
Abdomen + vagina	7.0
Abdomen + pelvis	23.0
Abdomen + pelvis + liver	14.0
Abdomen + brain	3.0
Vagina	19.0
Para-aortic nodes	3.0
Para-aortic nodes	19.0
Benign Cytology	
Lumbar spine	7.0
Lung	20.0
Abdomen	6.0
Brain	12.0
Pelvis	24.0
'Metastatic'	—

Table 6. Incidence of malignant peritoneal cytology.

Series	Date	All Stages			Stage I		
		Pos	Total	%	Pos	Total	%
Creasman [8]	1971	21	183	11.5			
Creasman [9]	1981						
Group 1					26	167	15.5
Group 2					23	~175	~13
Yazigi [10]	1983				10	93	11
Imachi [16]	1986	14	61	23	5	35	14.3
GOG [14]	1987				76	621	12.0
Harouny [12]	1988	72	340	21.3	47	276	17.1
Konski [11]	1988	19	134	14.2	14	127	11.0
Lurain [18]1	1988				30	157	19
Mazurka [17]	1988	34	280	12			
Total		160	99%	16.0	231	~1651	~14.0

Table 7. Histologic grade and myometrial invasion versus peritoneal cytology.

Series	Date	Grade				Myometrial invasion			
		1	2	3	P	Inner 1/3	Middle 1/3	Outer 1/3	P
Creasman [9]	1981	8/74*	15/63	3/30	NS	15/132	3/10	8/25	<.01
Yazigi [10]	1983	7/66	1/15	2/12	NS	6/44	1/35	3/14	NS
Imachi [16]	1986	4/28	8/22	2/11	NS	3/30	2/10	7/18	<.05
Harouny [12]	1988	10/104	18/103	13/41	<.01	24/185	5/28	12/35	<.01
Konski [11]	1988	6/70	10/54	3/10	NS	1/27	10/59	7/45	NS

includes only patients who had *no* preoperative therapy and may therefore be the best index. Correlation of clinical stage and incidence of malignant cytology in reported series is difficult because of small numbers. In contrast to the Indiana University/St. Vincent Hospital series [12], neither Yazigi et al. [10] nor Creasman et al. [9] identified a difference in malignant cytology between Stage IA and IB lesions. Imachi [16] and Konski [11] both demonstrated increasing malignant cytology with greater stage of disease, in agreement with our findings.

Histologic grade and myometrial depth have been evaluated by a number of authors whose findings are summarized in Table 7. Depth of myometrial invasion correlated with cytology status more often in these studies than did histologic grade.

Of clinical parameters, extrauterine spread of disease correlates most closely with malignant cytology. Positive washings were found in nine of 15 (60%) patients with adnexal spread and in 17 of 152 (11%) with negative adnexae, in the report of Creasman et al. [9]. This is in close agreement with our findings. Also consonant with findings of the Indiana University/St. Vincents Hospital series are the findings by Imachi et al. [16] of extrauterine disease in 64.3% of patients with malignant cytology and in only 12.8% of those with benign cytology. Mazurka et al. [17] noted that 18 of 34 (52.9%) patients with malignant cytology had other extrauterine spread, in contrast to nine of 246 (37%) of patients with negative washings. The Gynecologic Oncology Group [14] also noted extrauterine disease in 48% of patients with positive cytology and a 35% incidence of malignant cytology in those with extrauterine disease.

Metastases to pelvic or para-aortic lymph nodes occur in about 10% of all patients with Stage I disease. The reports of Creasman et al. [9] and the Gynecology Oncology Group [14] concur with the correlation between malignant cytology and pelvic or para-aortic lymph node metastases. The GOG study showed high correlations in both areas (P < 0.001) (Table 8).

Extrauterine spread in the form of pelvic, adnexal, or nodel metastases has an adverse effect upon disease-free and absolute survival in endometrial cancer. Since up to half of all patients with malignant peritoneal cytology have evidence of extrauterine spread, it is difficult to assess the independent effect of positive washings on survival. Our study suggests better outcome in patients with *surgical* Stage I disease if peritoneal cytology is benign; three of 11 patients with surgical Stage I disease died of recurrent cancer, compared to none of 62 with negative cytology. Yazigi et al. [10], Lurain et al. [18], and Konski et al. [11] suggest that malignant cytology has no effect upon survival; in the last series, however, recurrences were noted in 15% of patients with malignant washings and in only 5.2% of those with negative washings. Creasman and Rutledge [8] noted a significant survival difference (P = 0.003) at four years in patients of all stages depending upon peritoneal cytology. In clinical Stage I patients, Creasman et al. [9] subsequently demonstrated 90.1% disease-free survival rate in 141 patients with negative

Table 8. Correlation between lumph node metastases and peritoneal cytology.

Series	Date	Pelvic lymph nodes			Para-aortic lymph nodes		
		Pos	Neg	P	Pos	Neg	P
Creasman [9]	1981	11/17	15/150	<.001	8/11	13/123	<.001
Imachi [16]	1986	2/9	7/44	NS	4/11	0/46	<.01
GOG [14]	1987	19/57	56/555	<.0001	14/34	61/578	<.0001
Harouny [12]	1988	3/4	12/74		4/5	11/73	

cytology, compared to 66% disease-free survival in those with negative washings. The study of Imachi et al. [16] noted 92.3% and 75% survival in the same two groups of patients. We used the generalized Wilcoxon text to compare Kaplan–Meier estimates of survival and found significant differences based upon peritoneal cytology for disease-free survival in all stages (P < .001), as well as for survival in patients with clinical Stage I disease (P < .001).

Perhaps as significant as the apparent effect malignant cytology has upon recurrence rate and survival is the propensity for patients with positive washings to suffer relapse within the peritoneal cavity. Creasman et al. [9] reported that six of thirteen patients with positive cytology as the only manifestation of extrauterine spread died of abdominal carcinomatosis. Our findings were similar. Nine of 12 patients with clinical Stage I disease who suffered relapse had an abdominal component, compared to one of six patients with benign cytology.

Summary

The ultimate role played by peritoneal cytologic evaluation in endometrial cancer remains somewhat ill-defined. Proper assessment of peritoneal cytology as an independent risk factor awaits a prospective study in which patients with malignant peritoneal cytology and surgical Stage I lesions are not treated and survival is compared to controls with negative cytology. Such a study is unlikely to be done, given results available from retrospective analyses and the large number of patients needed to complete such a trial.

Whether therapy is needed and which type to use in patients with malignant cytology remain uncertain. Half of these patients will presumably require pelvic radiotherapy for adnexal, nodal, or other pelvic spread. Potish et al. [19] have advocated the use of whole-abdominal radiotherapy in such patients, with favorable results. In patients without extrauterine spread, Creasman et al. [9] have championed the postoperative use of intraperitoneal radioactive phosphate. They based their recommendation on survival results in a group of 23 patients with positive washings who were treated with intraperitoneal radioactive chromic phosphate. In this group, the recurrence rate was reduced, when compared to historic controls, to 13% (3/23), all of whom had extra-abdominal recurrences.

Soper et al. [15] confirmed the safety of postoperative radioactive chromic phosphate in doses of approximately 15 millicuries in patients with endometrial cancer. In their study of 65 patients, 56 had percutaneous catheter placement under local anesthesia after laparotomy. In one patient, the catheter could not be used because of poor distribution of the technetium Tc 99 m sulfur colloid tracer, and in a second subject, fever and peritoneal signs suggesting bowel perforation led to removal of the insertion catheter. No other significant problems were encountered in 48 patients treated with radioactive chromic phosphate without other therapy. In contrast, five of seventeen patients who received external pelvic radiotherapy in addition to radioactive chromic phosphate suffered bowel complications requiring surgical intervention. Two of these patients died of operative complications, suggesting that radioactive chromic phosphate cannot be safely combined with standard dose external radiotherapy.

In a retrospective series, Mazurka et al. [17] intimated that adjunctive chemotherapy might be useful in patients with malignant cytology, but such an approach is untested. A prospective randomized study of radioactive chromic phosphate, whole abdomen radiotherapy, or adjunctive chemotherapy versus no treatment in patients with malignant peritoneal cytology is clearly needed.

References

1. Saphir O, 1949. Cytologic diagnosis of cancer from pleural and peritoneal fluids. Am J Clin Pathol 19:309–314.
2. Keettel WC, Elkins HB, 1956. Experience with radioactive colloidal gold in the treatment of ovarian carcinoma. Am J Obstet Gynecol 71:553.
3. Morton DG, Moore, JG, Chang N, 1961. The clinical value of peritoneal lavage for cytologic examination. Am J Obstet Gynecol 81:1115.
4. Malkasian GP, Decker GG, Webb MJ, 1975. Histology of epithelial tumors of the ovary: Clinical usefulness and prognostic significance of the histologic classification and grading. Semin Oncol 2:191–201.
5. Keettel WC, Pixley EE, Buchsbaum HJ, 1974. Experience with peritoneal cytology in the management of gynecological malignancies. Am J Obstet Gynecol 120:174–182.
6. Keettel WC, Pixley EE, 1958. Diagnostic value of peritoneal washings. Clin Obstet Gynecol 1:592.
7. Marcus CC, 1962. Cytology of the peritoneal cavity in benign and malignant disease. Obstet Gynecol 120:710.
8. Creasman WT, Rutledge F, 1971. The prognostic value of peritoneal cytology in gynecologic malignant disease. Am J Obstet Gynecol 110:773–781.
9. Creasman WT, DiSaia PJ, Blessing J, Wilkinson RH, Johnston W, Weed JC, 1981. Prognostic significance of peritoneal cytology in patients with endometrial cancer and preliminary data concerning therapy with intraperitoneal radiopharmaceuticals. Am J Obstet Gynecol 141:921–929.

10. Yazigi R, Piver MS, Blumenson L, 1983. Malignant peritoneal cytology as prognostic indicator in stage I endometrial cancer. Obstet Gynecol 62:359–362.
11. Konski A, Poulter C, Keys H, et al., 1988. Absence of prognostic significance, peritoneal dissemination, and treatment advantage in endometrial cancer patients with positive peritoneal cytology. Int J Rad Oncol Bio Phys 4:49–55.
12. Harouny VR, Sutton GP, Clark SA, et al., 1988. The importance of peritoneal cytology in endometrial carcinoma. Obstet Gynecol 72:000.
13. Koss LG, 1979. Diagnostic cytology and its histopathologic basis. Philadelphia: Lippincott.
14. Creasman WT, Morrow CP, Bundy BN, et al., 1987. Surgical pathologic spread patterns of endometrial cancer. Cancer 60:2035–2041.
15. Soper JT, Creasman WT, Clarke–Pearson DL, et al., 1985. Intraperitoneal chromic phosphate P–32 suspension therapy of malignant peritoneal cytology in endometrial carcinoma. Am J Obstet Gynecol 153:191–196.
16. Imachi M, Tsukamoto N, Matsuyama T, et al., 1988. Peritoneal cytology in patients with endometrial carcinoma. Gynecol Oncol 30:76–86.
17. Mazurka JL, Krepart GV, Lotocki RJ, 1988. Prognostic significance of positive peritoneal cytology in endometrial carcinoma. Am J Obstet Gynecol 158:303–306.
18. Lurain JR, Rumsey NK, Schink JC, et al., 1988. Prognostic signifiance of positive peritoneal cytology in clinical stage I adenocarcinoma of the endometrium. (Meeting Abstract), American College of Obstetricians and Gynecologists Annual Clinical Meething, Boston.
19. Potish RA, Twiggs LB, Adcock LL, et al., 1985. Role of the whole abdominal radiation therapy in the management of endometrial cancer; prognostic importance of factors indicating peritoneal metastases. Gynecol Oncol 21:80–85.

4. The role of preoperative radiotherapy in the treatment of carcinoma of the endometrium

Nina Einhorn

Introduction

The role of irradiation in the management of endometrial carcinoma has been well recognized during this century. In the beginning, the irradiation was used only as therapeutic modality, but with improved surgical techniques, anaesthetic capabilities as well as improved management of cardiovascular disorders, the combination of irradiation and surgery became the treatment of choice in the late 1940s, and it persisted as a method of choice for next three decades. During the late 1970s and early 1980s, a new school advocating primary surgery developed, two basic factors favored this new approache: (1) the disadvantage of radiation exposure to personnel, and (2) the possibility of tailoring the postoperative treatment by the staging laparotomy.

To assess preoperative radiotherapy treatment in endometrial carcinoma, it is necessary to make an objective study of the advantages and disadvantages of the method and to try in an objective way to determine when preoperative radiotherapy will benefit the patient. Unfortunately, there have been very few scientifically designed clinical trials that randomly compare large numbers of patients with endometrial carcinoma. Most of the results are based on retrospective studies. Nevertheless, many of them have been made on large patient populations, with sincere attempts to draw the right conclusions.

The questions mostly debated today are (1) the sequence of irradiation and surgery: whether the irradiation should be given pre- or postoperatively; (2) the technique of irradiation given preoperatively; intracavitary versus external; (3) the choice of intracavitary treatment: Heyman packings, versus tandem and ovoid application; (4) low-dose versus high-dose rate intracavitary treatment; and (5) the interval between preoperative irradiation and surgery.

Preoperative versus Postoperative Irradiation

This seems to be the most controversial issue to be considered. Of course, if controversy is assumed from the beginning, the answer can never be

E. Surwit and D. Alberts (eds.), ENDOMETRIAL CANCER. Copyright © 1989.
Kluwer Academic Publishers, Boston. All rights reserved.

definite. There are, however, many studies advocating the usefulness of preoperative irradiation in a large proportion of patients with endometrial carcinoma. It becomes evident that the selection of patients suitable for preoperative irradiation should be based on the prognostic factors.

One of the most important prognostic factors well-recognized today is the grade of the tumor. With the new morphologic techniques, we may assume that in the future this will be better defined by other measures, such as DNA content. Today, the most established method of recognizing the different morphologic changs is still by defining the differentiation grade of the tumor. In a large number of studies, the well differentiated tumors have shown less ability to penetrate the myometrium or to metastasize to the lymph nodes. By now several studies have also documented the fact that the well differentiated tumor in Stage I can equally well be primarily operated, with results as good as with preoperative radiotherapy [1].

In selecting patients for preoperative irradiation the rationales are as follows: (1) the irradiated cancer cells are less clonogenic and have a lower ability to be implanted by surgical manipulations; (2) the tumor shrinkage promotes a better surgical procedure and sterlilization of peripheral tumor extension renders non-resectable tumors resectable; (3) the dose distribution given by intracavitary treatment influences nodal metastases; and (4) the amount of residual tumor will be greater in the non-preoperatively treated group, and a larger number of patients would need postoperative irradiation, which creates greater morbidity and greater complication rates.

What is the evidence to justify these postulates? Milagros [2] has reported a five-year survival rate of 77% for patients with viable-appearing residual tumors and 94% for patients without residual tumors, following preoperative intracavitary radiotherapy.

McCabe and Sagerman [3] observed 14% failures when residual tumor was present and only 3% when there was no residual tumor.

Macasaet et al. [4], as well as Komaki [5] and Toonkel [6], demonstrated a decreased survival associated with residual deep endometrial penetration, as compared with a lesser extent of residual tumor. Toonkel found an 83% five-year survival for patients with no residual tumors, 81% for patients with superficial myometrial penetration, and a 57% survival rate for patients with deep myometrial residual penetration. In the Macasaet material, two treatment methods were identified: radiotherapy followed by operation, and operation followed by radiotherapy. There was a clear correlation between the occurrence of residual tumor and the survival rate. Only 6% of the patients with no residual tumor died of their disease, compared with 28% of the group of patients with residual tumor. The patients that did not have residual tumor but who died of cancer had distant metastases but no evidence of pelvic recurrence.

Komaki, in his work describing the influence of preoperative irradiation on failures of endometrial carcinoma, has shown a highly significant statistical difference in the survival rates for patients with residual and no residual tumor. Patients with no residual tumor had a five-year survival of 96%, as compared with 65% for those who had residual tumor.

Chung et al. [7] have observed that the incidence of deep myometrial invasion in the preoperatively treated group was 6%, which could be compared with 28% for deep myometrial invasion in the postoperatively treated group.

Wharam et al. [8] have shown in a large study that in Grade II patients in the preoperatively treated group only 4% developed recurrent disease, as compared with 18% of the patients who developed recurrence in the primarily operated group with postoperative irradiation. As for the Grade III group, there was a 41% recurrence rate in the preoperatively treated group, compared with 62% in the postoperatively treaed group. They pointed out that the group operated primarily without preoperatively given irradiation clearly had a significantly higher risk of recurrent disease than if they had been given preoperative irradiation. There could be some bias in the selection made for postoperative irradiation. But even taking this fact into consideration, the authors do not feel that a randomized trial should be recommended for Grade III patients, since the difference in survival between pre- and postoperative irradiation was so great.

In a large survey made by the Canadian Association of Radiologists [9] describing the treatment results of a total of 2,719 patients of all stages treated during 1973–1977, the five-year survival in the preoperatively treated group was 85.9% and in the postoperatively treated group 81.6%, with a complication rate in the first group of 3.8% and in the second of 11.9%. They concluded that it is safer to give preoperative rather than postoperative treatment. It largely avoids administering external beam radiotherapy, with its potentially high complication rate and no benefit in extended survival. The same conclusion could be drawn from the work of Surwit et a. [10], which compared a non-selected patient population treated in two different ways in the Stockholm-region: one group was operated primarily independent of the grade and stage of disease, and the other group of Grade II and III patients were given treatment with preoperative irradiation. For the Grade II group, the survival rate was similar, 89% for the preoperatively treated patients and 91% for postoperatively treated patients. But for Grade III, there was a significant difference in the survival rate for the preoperatively treated patients (90%) and for postoperatively treated patients (75%). However, what was most important in this study was the difference in the number of patients with deep myometrial invasion in the primary surgically treated group, which consequently had to be subjected to postoperative external irradiation.

In a 1984 work by Bedwinek and coworkers [11], the residual tumor had a high influence on the survival rate, resulting in a highly significant difference in the survival rate for patients with no residual tumor and those with residual tumor, 93% and 67% five-year survival respectively. This paper considered only patients with Grade III tumors. The authors also suggested that preoperative treatment, with good uterine packings and intravaginal treatment, is more effective in preventing pelvic recurrences than are postoperative implants, which treat only the vaginal apex, and that the pelvic recurrence rate, which had been maximally reduced by the preoperative uterine and vaginal implant, could not be further reduced by postoperative irradiation.

In Bedwinek's paper, a highly significant difference in survival was observed for different milligram hour (mgh) applications in the uterus. Thirty-eight% of the patients with less than 2,500 mgh had pelvic failures, as compared with 8% for patients for whom 2,500–3,500 mgh were delivered and 0% for patients for whom more than 3,500 mgh was delivered. Their conclusion was that in spite of the idea that Heyman packings ought to be superfluous when a hysterectomy is also performed, it seems that there is a strong inverse correlation between the failure rate and the number of mgh to the uterine cavity. Their conclusion was that the intrauterine irradiation would appear to be a very important surgical adjunct, at least for Grade III lesions. This also influences the incidence of both pelvic and distant metastases. The rationale behind this observation is that the uterine implant diminishes the exfoliation of cells from the uterine serosa either before or during surgery.

In retrospective analyses made by Jazy and coworkers [12], the preoperative radiotherapy group had only a 4% incidence of deep myometrial invasion versus 31% in the postoperatively treated group. Of interest in this study was that in the preoperative group the depth of infiltration was not correlated to the differentiation grade. The patients treated with preoperative irradiation had an increased survival rate both for five and ten year observation periods.

Some authors point out that preoperative irradiation also influences the incidence of positive pelvic nodes found later in surgery [13, 14], suggesting that a low-dose irradiation delivered to the pelvic wall has some influence on the nodal metastases and that this influences the survival rate.

Preoperative brachytherapy versus external therapy

In 1977, Landgren and co-authors described the results of preoperative irradiation, comparing intracavitary radium either with Heyman packings or tandem and ovoids to preoperative external irradiation plus diminished radium treatment. They concluded that the pelvic tumor control was best when radium alone was utilized, regardless of the stage, grade, or specific histology of the tumor.

A very important randomized study comparing preoperative intracavitary treatment with preoperative external irradiation was reported by Weigensberg in 1984 [15]. FIGO Stage I patients were randomly allocated, prior to hysterectomy, either to a single implant with Heyman capsules and/or tandem and ovoids or external MeV irradiation. The five-year survival rate for the brachytherapy group was 80%, compared with 70% for the group treated with external irradiation. The ten-year acturial disease-free survivals were 67% and 59% respectively. Major complicaions occurred with equal frequency in both groups, but minor complications were seen more frequently in the external bean group. The conclusion from this paper was that intracavitary irradiation seems to be superior to external beam irradiation, in terms of a higher disease-free survival, lower frequency of recurrence, and fewer complications.

In Komaki's work from 1984, there was a difference in the survival rate between the patients treated with external and intracavitary treatment, external treatment alone, or intracavitary treatment alone. Patients with external plus intracavitary treatment had a five-year survival rate of 83%, compared with 64% for the intracavitary group. Due to small sample sizes these differences were not statistically significant.

Timing between preoperative irradiation and surgery

During the last decade a trend to shorten the time between preoperative irradiation and surgery has developed. It was started in 1969 at the M.D. Anderson Hospital, where patients with cancer of the endometrium limited to the uterus were treated with one radium insert followed by extrafascial hysterectomy at the same admission. Analyses in 1977 showed that only one out of 43 patients who could be followed died of cancer, and one died from complications. In a work described by Stokes [15], it was shown that the presence of residual tumor implied a significantly worse prognosis among the patients who received no preoperative irradiation *or* preoperative irradiation followed by immediate hysterectomy. In the patients undergoing hysterectomy four to six weeks after irradiation, myometrial invasion was described. Myometrial invasion greater than one-third was noted only in 1%, 5%, and 6% for Grades I, II, and III respectively. For patients with immediate hysterectomy following preoperative implant or with postoperative irradiation, deep myometrial invasion was noted in 29%, 41%, and 33% for the respective grades. Among the patients who did not receive preoperative irradiation or who underwent hysterectomy immediately after preoperative implant, greater than one-third myometrial invasion was associated with a significantly reduced survival rate.

In 1986, Delmore et al. [16] published the M.D. Anderson Hospital experience on two versus one radium application with presurgery times of six to eight weeks and two to three days respectively. The patients who had two treatments before surgery had a five-year survival rate of 91.4%, which compared with the one radium treatment group, which had an 84.2% survival rate. The author claims that the short time interval method with one radium insert is more cost effective.

Preoperative high-dose contra low-dose irradiation

There is only one study that compares the high-dose afterloading technique (cathetron) with low-dose intracavitary irradiation. The study was carried out in Finland by Taina and coworkers [18]. In their work, no statistical difference was found between the two treatment groups with regard to early or late postoperative complications, and no difference in survival could be observed for the two groups.

Techniques

Intrauterine Brachy methods, Heyman packings

The method was first described by James Heyman in 1935 [20] and also by Kottmeier in 1959 [21] and by Joelsson [22], and was modified as a semi-afterloading method by Norman Simon. This technique is still used as a main method for inoperable patients with endometrial carcinoma and is also used preoperatively for the high-grade endometrial cancer patients, as well as for Stage II of all grades. The method is based on fractionated irradiation and, in general, two courses with a three week interval are given if hysterectomy is planned to follow. A third packing is performed in patients where surgery is considered to be contraindicated. In these cases curettage is performed three months later.

The method is characterized by an attempt to insert as many capsules as possible into the corpus cavity in order to distend the cavity and reduce the thickness of the uterine wall. A reduction in the wall thickness to one-third of its normal values will greatly increase the dose to the serous surface. Two packings should deliver an estimated tumorcidal dose of 60–100 Gy with a dose of 30 Gy 1.5 cm from the applicators. The Heyman capsules are usually loaded with 35–48 Co^{137} equivalent to 14–19 mg radium. Through the work done by Joelsson et al., it is estimated that the mean dose to the surface of the corporal level of the uterus during one treatment course varies between 10–15 Gy but at the circumference ranges between 6–50 Gy. Using the same experiment set-up and central cylindric applicator, it was found that the surface dose was considerably decreased with a central applicator.

The Heyman applicators are in stainless steel and have to be applied manually into the uterus cavity. The Norman Simon applicators are in plastic material and can be afterloaded after the primary packing, which promotes a quicker application of the sources. Usually the doses to the bladder and rectum are measured after application, but dosimetry to bladder and rectum can equally well be achieved by taking X-ray pictures of the Norman Simon applicators before the sources are inserted and by calculating the dosimetry from the X-ray films.

58

Recently, a totally remote afterloading system has been developed by the Selectron Corporation in the Netherlands, whereby a Heyman packing system can be introduced completely automatically into the uterine cavity.

Intravaginal intracavitary treatment

Essentially all studies today agree that the irradiation of the vagina reduces the recurrence rate, which varies between 7% and 20% and which is reduced to 1% when intracavity vaginal treatment is given. This treatment can be given in association with the preoperative intrauterine irradiaiton, if preferred. The vaginal treatment can be given either as vaginal cylinder, giving even irradiation to the distal part of the vagina. Most authors today would consider that irradiation of the upper vagina will adequately irradiate the high-risk surface. A vaginal mucosa-surface dose in the range 60–70 Gy has proved adequate to reduce recurrence to less than 1% [23, 24].

In the Stockholm technique using the vaginal cylinder and radium source, the aim of the irradiation was to give approximately 18 Gy 1 cm from the vaginal mucosa. By using the remote afterloading system with cesium sources, the dose has now been modified to 13 Gy at 1 cm distance.

External irradiation

When external irradiation is used without any intracavitary treatment preoperatively, 30–40 gray is usually given over three to five weeks, using either a two-field or a four-field technique. The two-field technique can be given either by a portal of 15 × 15 cm or by a field with a lower limit of foramina obturatoria to an upper limit of between L4 and L5 and laterally 1 cm outside the pelvic cavity. For the four-field technique, the lateral field would normally be 9 × 15 cm and the posterior anterior fields 15 × 15 cm.

Conclusions

Preoperative irradiaton is at present a controversial issue. The advocates of these methods are pointing out the differences in survival for patients with tumor residual, documented in many studies, as well as that the morbidity is reduced because the requirement for postoperative irradiation is minimized through preoperative irradiation. On the other hand, the advocates for postoperative treatment claim that it is possible to tailor the treatment after the surgical staging laparatomy. Today, we do not have a clear answer to these two schools of thought. However, if preoperative irradiation is to be given and probably it should be given to the poorer prognostic groups , high quality radiotherapy is essential if good results are to be expected.

References

1. Karlstedt K, 1968. Carcinoma of the uterine corpus. Acta Radiologica, Suppl No 282.
2. Milagros M, Brigati D, Boyce J, et al., 1980. The significance of residual disease after radiotherapy in endometrial carcinoma, clinicopathologic correlation. Am J Obstet Gynecol 138:557.
3. McCabe J, Sagerman RH, 1979. Treatment of endometrial cancer in a regional radiation therapy center. Cancer 43:1052–1057.
4. Macasaet M, Brigati D, Boyce J, Nicasri A, Waxman M, Nelson J, Fruchter R, 1980. The significance of residual disease after radiotherapy in endometrial carcinoma: Clinicopthologic correlation. Am J Obstet Gynecol 138:557–563.
5. Komaki R, Cox JD, Hartz A, Wilson JF, Greenberg M, 1984. Influence of preoperative irradiation on failures of endometrial carcinoma with high risk of lymph node metastasis. Am J Clin Oncol 7:661–668.
6. Toonkel LM, Fix I, Jacobson LH, Bamberg N, Wallach CB, 1984. Myometrial penetration of endometrial carcinoma as a prognostic factor for patients receiving pre- or postoperative radiation therapy. Am J Clin Oncol 7:669–673.
7. Chung CK, Stryker JA, Nahhas WA, Mortel R, 1981. The role of adjunctive radiotherapy for stage I endometrial carcinoma: Preoperative vs postoperative irradiation. J Radiation Oncology Biol Phys 7:1429–1435.
8. Wharam MD, Phillips TL, Bagshaw MA, 1976. The role of radiation therapy in clinical stage I carcinoma of the endometrium. J Radiation Oncology Biol Phys 1:1081–1089.
9. Starreveld AA, Shankowsky HA, Koch M, 1987. Canadian Association of Radiologists: Treatment results in 2719 patients with carcinoma of the endometrium 1973–1977. J Can Assoc Radiol 38:96–105.
10. Surwit EA, Joelsson I, Einhorn N, 1981. Adjunctive radiation therapy in the mangement of stage I cancer of the endometrium. Obstet Gynecol 58:590–595.
11. Bedwinek J, Galakatos A, Camel M, Kao M-S, Stokes S, Perez C, 1984. Stage I, grade III adenocarcinoma of the endometrium treated with surgery and irradiation. Cancer 54: 40–47.
12. Jazy FK, Shehata WM, Dobrogorski OJ, Alamin K, Schmidt RTF. 1983. Pre-operative versus postoperative irradiation in stage I carcinoma of the endometrium. Clinical Oncol 9:281–288.
13. Creasman WT, Boronow RC, Morrow CP, DiSaia PJ, Blessing J, 1976. Adenocarcinoma of the endometrium: Its metastatic lymph node potential. Gynecol Oncol 4:239.
14. Landgren RD, Fletcher GH, Galager HS, Declos L, Wharton JT, 1977. Treatment failure sites according to irradiation technique and histology in patients with endometrial cancer. Cancer 40:131–135.
15. Weigensberg IJ, 1984. Preoperative radiation therapy in stage I endometrial adenocarcinoma. Cancer 53:242–247.
16. Stokes S, Bedwinek J, Kao M-S, Camel HM, Perez CA, 1986. Treatment of stage I adenocarcinoma of the endometrium by hysterectomy and adjuvant irradiation: A retrospective analysis of 304 patients. J Radiation Oncol Biol Phys 12:339–344.
17. Delmore JE, Wharton JT, Hamberger AD, Saul PB, Gershensson DM, Copeland LJ, 1986. Preoperative radiotherapy for early endometrial carcinoma. Gynecol Oncol 28:34–40.
18. Prem KA, Adcock LL, Okagaki T, Jones TK, 1979. The evolution of a treatment program for adenocarcinoma of the endometrium. Am J Obstet Gynecol 13:803–812.
19. Taina E, Mäenpää J, Erkkola R, Kilkku P, 1987. Influence of preoperative intracavitary high (Co60, cathetron) and low dose-rate (radium) irradiation on surgical difficulties and postsurgical morbidity in patients with uterine carcinoma. Ann Chir et Gyn 76:202:72–75.
20. Heyman J, 1935. The co-called Stockholm method and the results of treatment of uterine cancer at the Radiumhemmet. Acta Radiol 16:129.

21. Kottmeier HL, 1959. Carcinoma of the corpus uteri: diagnosis and therapy. Am J Obstet Gynecol 78:1127.
22. Joelsson I, Sandri A, Kottmeir HL, 1973. Carcinoma of the uterine corpus. Acta Radiol, suppl 334.
23. Underwood PB, Lutz MH, Kreutner A, Miller MC, Johnson RD, 1977. Carcinoma of the endometrium. Radiation followed immediately by operation. Am J Obstet Gynecol 128:86.
24. DePalo G, Kenda R, Andreola S, Luciani L, Musumecia J, Rilke F, 1982. Endometrial Carcinoma: Stage I. Obstet Gynecol 60:225.

5. Radiotherapy in the management of nodal and peritoneal metastases

Roger A. Potish

Introduction

Endometrial carcinoma clinically confined to the uterus is all too infrequently cured, despite virtually complete control of pelvic tumor by contemporary surgical and radiotherapeutic techniques. Although selected series have achieved somewhat better results, five-year survival rates worldwide are 75% for Stage I and 58% for Stage II endometrial carcinomas and have not substantially improved over the past few decades, despite high rates of operability and widespread utilization of pelvic adjuvant radiation therapy [1]. Occult peritoneal and lymph node metastases are responsible for a major fraction of recurrences. Although earlier studies had hinted at an appreciable rate of nodal and peritoneal spread in early endometrial carcinoma, its importance was not fully proven until the data of the Gynecologic Oncology Group became available [2, 3]. Simultaneously, information was generated concerning the efficacy of radiation for treatment of such metastases [4, 5]. Perhaps the next decade will witness an improvement in cure, as appropriate surgical staging and extended field radiation therapy techniques gain greater acceptance.

Nodal metastases

A substantial incidence of nodal metastases has been documented for Stage I endometrial cancer by the Gynecologic Oncology Group, and it is likely that higher stages have even greaer metastatic rates [2, 3, 6]. Selective pelvic and periaortic lymphadenectomies were performed in 621 patients undergoing total abdominal hysterectomy, bilateral salpingo-oophorectomy, and peritoneal fluid sampling [2]. Overall, 11% had positive pelvic and/or periaortic lymph node metastases: 6% with positive pelvics and negative periaortics, 3% with positive pelvics and positive periaortics, and 2% with positive periaortics and negative pelvics. Pelvic node metastates were found in 7% of Stage IA and 13% of Stage IB. Periaortic node metastases were found in 3% of Stage IA and 8% of Stage IB. As grade increaseed from 1 to

3, positive pelvic nodes rose from 3% to 18%, and positive periaortic nodes rose from 2% to 11%. Similarly, as depth of myometrial invasion increased from none to deep, pelvic node positivity rose from 1% to 25%, and periaortic node positivity rose from 1% to 17%. The highest rates of nodal metastases were found in high grade lesions with deep myometrial invasion. Of 73 clinically occult Stage II endometrial cancers, there were 20% positive pelvic and 14% positive aortic nodes [3]. Collected series of Stage II endometrial cancers, presumably with a larger proportion of gross cervical lesions, had a 36% pelvic node metastatic rate [6].

The mere demonstration of node metastases is of little importance if they can not be cured. Node metastases throughout the body can be satisfactorily controlled with moderate doses of radiation. This was first proven for such clinically accessible areas as adenocarcinomas of the breast and squamous cell carcinomas of the upper respiratory and digestive tracts. Subclinical lymph node disease could almost always be controlled with 50 Gy in five weeks with conventional 2 Gy fraction size [7]. Half of 1–3 cm neck nodes could be controlled with this dose, and greater doses controlled larger nodes with greater probability [7]. Some 40% of women with periaortic node metastases from squamous cell carcinomas or adenocarcinomas of the cervix can be cured with radiation with 45 to 50 Gy of extened field radiation [5]. This same dose has been demonstrated to improve survival in women with nodal metastases from squamous cell carcinoma of the vulva [8]. Thus, it is not surprising that endometrial carcinomas spread to nodal areas can be cured with radiation therapy.

The University of Minnesota experience in the management of nodal metastases of endometrial carcinoma is representative of modern radiotherapy [4, 5]. Periaortic radiation was given with daily fraction sizes of 1.50–1.75 Gy with 8–9 cm wide anterior and posterior parallel-opposed beams extending from the top of standard pelvic fields to the level of theT–10 to T–12 vertebral bodies. Periaortic dose ranged from 45 to 51 Gy. Pelvic nodes were boosted with pelvic portals containing a midline block. Pelvic fields extended from the bottom of the obturator foramen to the level of the 4th or 5th lumbar vertebral body and 1–2 cm lateral to the bony pelvis. Cobalt and linear accelerator beams (4–24 MV) were used, the majority of with 10–MV photons. Cesium or radium were used for intracavitary Fletcher applications.

Of six patients with biopsy-proven metastases confined to pelvic nodes, four survived free of disease at five years. In 15 women with biopsy-proven periaortic metastases, with or without concurrent pelvic node metastases, the actuarial observed and relapse-free five-year survival probabilities were .40 and .42 respectively. Of eight sites of first recurrence, four were abdominal, one was abdominal and hematogenous, one was pelvic, one was supraclavicular and one was hematogenous. No patient who relapsed was salvaged. There were no statistically significant survival differences by age, stage, grade, histopathologic category, or bulk of nodal tumor, but the relatively small sample size may well have masked such differences. Acute and chronic tolerance were both satisfactory; only one patient developed a small bowel obstruction and she did not require surgical intervention. Acceptable complication rates have been observed elsewhere, as have survival rates approaching 40% in women with periaortic metastases [3, 9, 10]. The survival of women with pelvic node metastases may be somewhat greater, but this is not well established in the current literature [3].

Malignant cells in the peritoneal fluid

Some 12% of women with Stage I endometrial cancer have malignant cells in their peritoneal fluid at initial diagnosis. [2]. Half of the women with malignant cells in the peritoneal fluid have no other demonstrable extrauterine disease. One quarter have pelvic nodal metastases; one fifth have periaortic nodal metastases. Conversely, one third of women with other extrauterine disease have malignant cells in the peritoneal fluid. As grade rises from 1 to 3, the malignant cytology rates goes from 6% to 17% [3]. As myometrial invasion deepens from none to outer third, the incidence of malignant cytology increases from 6% to 17%. As for nodal metastases, the highest rate of malignant cells in the peritoneal fluid occurs with the combination of high grade and deep myometrial invasion.

There are two successful forms of management of malignant cells in the peritoneal fluid. The intraperitoneal instillation of radioactive isotopes is associated with survivals of 89% in clinical Stage I and of 94% in otherwise surgical Stage I endometrial carcinoma [11]. While this therapy is quite effective for tumor control, 29% of patients who also received pelvic radiation developed severe bowel damage. The toxicity of combining radioactive isotopes and external beam therapy has been shown in a number of series [12–14]. Thus, the use of radioactive isotopes should be limited to patients who do not require additional external beam therapy.

The University of Minnesota has utilized open field whole abdominal radiation therapy to treat malignant cells in the peritoneal fluid [15, 16]. The entire abdominal cavity received 20 Gy with daily fraction size of 1 Gy. Abdominal field height extended from above the dome of the diaphragm to the bottom of the obturator foramen and lateral beyond the peritoneal fat stripe. Fluoroscopy was used to ensure that there was at least 1 cm of margin above the diaphragm. No renal or hepatic shielding was used. All patients were scheduled to receive external beam pelvic boosts, except one woman who developed a small bowel obstruction before initiation of radiotherapy. External beam boosts to the pelvic ranged from 19 to 30 Gy. In women with nodal metastases, periaortic node boost doses ranged from 24 to 30 Gy with daily fraction size of 1.50 to 1.75 Gy. Cesium or radium was also utilized.

The five-year relapse-free rate was 73%, and the abdomen was the most common site of failure [15, 16]. Too few patients were available to analyze associated prognsotic factors in sufficient detail. Both acute and chronic morbidity were satisfactory, with 4% of patients treated with this technique developing small bowel obstruction. Although survival was high and morbidity was low, other series have reported good survival despite no treatment of the peritoneal cavity with either external beam radiation or intraperitoneal isotopes [17, 18]. One study did show a 28% survival benefit from the use of radioactive isotopes, but it was not randomized [19].

Gross intraperitoneal spread

Some 6% of women with Stage I endometrial carcinoma have gross intraperitoneal metastases found at initial surgery [2]. Half of the women with such spread also have pelvic nodal metastases, and one quarter have periaortic nodal metastases. If both deep myometrial invasion and gross intraperitoneal disease are present, two thirds are associated with pelvic node metastases and one third with periaortic node metastases.

Radiation therapy has only limited efficacy in the management of gross peritoneal disease. The University of Minnesota experience with use of whole abdominal radiation did not initially report any five-year survivals [15]. As more patients have been treated, the five-year relapse-free rate has increased to 31% [16]. Because of incomplete operative reporting, it was not possible to stratify such patents by extent or by initial or residual disease. However, the moving-strip whole abdominal techniques showed a substantial effect of tumor bulk. If residual disease was no greater than 2 cm, the five-year survival rate was 80% [20]. All patients with more extensive residual disease died from cancer. The cure rates from open field and moving strip radiation therapy are similar to those expected for epithelial carcinoma of the ovary [21]. The high rate of associated lymph node metastases may make women with gross endometrial intraperitoneal metastases even more difficult to cure [2]. Nevertheless, as with ovarian cancer, surgical debulking may be of substantial benefit.

Adnexal metastases

Metastases to the tube or ovary occur in 5% of women with Stage I cancer [2]. If adnexal involvement is present, one third are associated with pelvic node metastases and one fifth with aortic node metastases. When treated with abdominal and pelvic radiation therapy, relapse-free survival was 82% at five years [15, 16]. This is similar to that expected from the use of radiation in epithelial cancer of the ovary [21]. However, similar results have been reported with radiation delivered solely to the pelvis for adnexal metastases [22, 23]. As with malignant cells in the peritoneal fluid, the prognostic significance of adnexal metastases remains unclear.

Papillary serous histology

Papillary histology has emerged as a possible predictor of peritoneal spread. One study documented a 50% relapse rate in patients with pathologic Stage I papillary serous endometrial carcinoma [24], which morphologically closely resembles ovarian papillary serous adenocarcinoma. These lesions are associated with deeper mymometial invasion and more upper abdominal failures than are endometrioid adenocarcinomas. Adjuvant upper abdominal radiation or chemotherapy has been proposed whenever this histologic subtype has been identified [25].

Recommendations

It is clear that 40% of women with periaortic lymph node metastases can be cured with extended field radiation therapy [3–5, 9, 10]. This survival rate will be somewhat higher in the absence of and lower in the presence of peritoneal metastases [3, 5]. Isolated pelvic node metastases may have an even greater chance of cure [3, 4]. Thus, nodal sampling should be performed in all women with endometrial cancer, unless precluded by their overall medical condition. Even though the nodal metastatic rate is low for low grade and minimal myometrial invasion, some metastases do occur. In addition, it is not uncommon for the final pathology report to reveal deeper myometrial invasion than clinically suspected, occult cervical involvement, or higher grade than at dilatation and curretage. The importance of adequate lymph node sampling is underlined by the fact that over 90% of such spread occurs in grossly normal nodes [2]. The morbidity of extended field radiation is low enough to consider elective nodal radiation for such risk factors as high grade and deep myometrial invastion if nodes are not sampled [4, 5].

The presence of malignant cells in the peritoneal fluid has an uncertain biologic and prognostic significance. Survivals higher than 70% have been reported with whole abdominal external beam therapy, with intraperitoneal radioactive isotopes, and with no treatment of the peritoneal cavity [11, 15–18]. All series have small numbers of patients, and pathologic criteria of malignancy may vary. The one study showing a survival advantage to intraperitoneal isotopes was not randomized [19]. Nevertheless, it is difficult for the clinician and the patient to ignore the presence of malignancy beyond conventional surgical and radiation fields. A randomized clinical trial is necessary to prove the need for treatment of this spread pattern, but a very large sample size will be necessary in view of the small survival difference to be expected, as indicated by the data on patients not treated for such metastases. In the interim, it remains reasonable to treat the abdomen with external beam or radioactive isotopes. If, however, adjuvant pelvic radiation is used for other risk factors, the morbidity of concurrent intraperitoneal isotopes is substantial [11–14, 19]. Such patients should be treated solely with external beam and intracavitary techniques, described previously [15].

Gross intraperitoneal metastases confer an ominous prognosis unless they can be reduced to less than 2 cm [15, 16, 20]. In ovarian cancer, abdomino-pelvic radiation achieved five-year survival rates of 80% with no gross residual tumor, 56% with residual tumor less than 2 cm, and 10% with residual tumor greater than or equal to 2 cm [21]. These results are mirrored by the open field and moving strip abdominal radiation techniques [16, 20]. Although, as with ovarian cancer, it is possible that readily debulkable tumors might be less biologically aggressive and therefore would not be helped by debulking, the limited radiation doses achievable in the upper abdomen would argue in favor of vigorous debulking. If there is less than 2 cm of residual tumor, external beam radiation to the abdomen offers an excellent probability of cure [20]. Microscopic peritoneal metastases have also been successfully treated with intraperitoneal isotopes [26]. If more extensive disease remains, one option is to treat such patients with the same cytotoxic agents utilized in the management of ovarian cancer. Unfortunate-ly, their prognosis will probably be no better than women with suboptimal ovarian cancer. Thus, experimental therapy should be considered, although there will likely be a few long-term survivors with conventional radiotherapy or chemotherapy.

Adnexal metastases have an excellent prognosis when treated with whole abdominal radiation therapy [15, 16]. Nevertheless, as with malignant cells in the peritoneal fluid, the prognostic meaning of such spread remains unclear [22, 23]. Although good results have been reported with pelvic radiation alone following surgery, it seems prudent to utilize whole abdom-inal therapy in view of its low morbidity. Another rationale for the use of whole abdominal and pelvic radiation is the frequent difficulty in distin-guishing metastases to the ovary from a primary ovarian tumor; radiation therapy is quite effective regardless of the site of origin, whereas cytotoxic chemotherapy has not been proven to be beneficial for endometrial carci-noma in the adjuvant setting. Still, a randomized clinical trial is necessary to definitively answer the necessity of such therapy.

Papillary serous histology also awaits a randomized clinical trial to de-monstate the need for and efficacy of adjuvant radiation and chemotherapy. This entity also needs more universal pathologic definition. Incidence rates for this subtype range from 4% or less to 10%, presumably reflecting varying criteria for diagnosis [24, 25]. At the University of Minnesota, papillary serous histology is treated with pelvic radiation, unless evidence of peritoneal spread is documented. If peritoneal spread is demonstrated, it is reasonable to treat the entire abdominal cavity. If more than 2 cm gross residual peritoneal disease is present, chemotherapy or experimental ther-apy is indicated. Until a definitive answer is found, elective abdominal radiation is also a viable option for papillary serous histology without proven extrauterine spread.

Multiple extrauterine risk factors confer a worse prognosis than do single risk factors [3]. This is particularly true for the combination of nodal and peritoneal metastases [5]. Nevertheless, radiation therapy to the appropriate areas still offers the hope of cure for at least a fraction of such women. Hematogenous metastases remain an important site of failure, and these will become even more important as extended field radiation controls an ever greater proportion of peritoneal and nodal metastases. In addition, substantial numbers of abdominal recurrences develop despite the most optimal use of radiotherapy. Thus the next steps in the cure of women with endometrial cancer most likely will involve effective systemic therapy, although such modalities as intraperitoneal chemotherapy and hyperfractionated radiotherapy may add to the probability of abdominal control.

Until more effective therapy is developed, the cornerstone of improved management of women with early endometrial cancer is identification and treatment of extrauterine metastases. A full 25% of women with Stage I endometrial carcinoma do not survive five years following diagnosis [1]. It is probably not coincidental that 22% of Stage I cancers have occult extrauterine metastases at initial diagnosis [2]. This can be further subdivided into 6% with and 16% without gross peritoneal disease. Few of the former can be cured, but a majority of the latter are potentially curable with extended radiation fields. Thus, it is realistic to expect a 5% to 10% overall survival improvement by the use of appropriately extended nodal and abdominal radiation fields. While this will not dramatically increase the chance of cure, it will be very worthwhile for the individual women who are cured, with little increase in morbidity. Issues still to be resolved concern the necessity of extended field radiation in various peritoneal spread patterns and the development of effective adjuvant and salvage systemic therapy.

References

1. Pettersson F, Kolstad P, Ludwig H, Ulfelder H, 1985. Annual report on the results of treatment in gynecologic cancer, Vol 19, Stockholm, Trycker: Baider, pp. 123–205.
2. Creasman WT, Morrow CP, Bundy BN, Homesley HD, Graham JE, Heller PB, 1987. Surgical pathologic spread patterns of endometrial cancer: A Gynecologic Oncology Group study. Cancer 60:2035–2041.
3. Morrow CP, Creasman WT, Homesley H, Yordan E, Park R, Bundy B, 1986. Recurrence of endometrial carcinoma as a function of extended surgical staging data (a Gynaecological Oncology Group study). In Gynaecological Oncology (Morrow CP, Smart GE, eds). Berlin: Springer, pp. 147–153.
4. Potish RA, Twiggs LB, Adcock LL, Savage JE, Levitt SH, Prem KA, 1985. Paraaortic lymph node radiotherapy in cancer of the uterine corpus. Obstet Gynecol 65:251–256.
5. Potish RA, 1987. Radiation therapy of periaortic node metastases in cancer of the uterine cervix and endometrium. Radiology 165:567–570.
6. Morrow CP, DiSaia PJ, Townsend DE, 1973. Current management of endometrial carcinoma. Obstet Gynecol 42:399–406.
7. Fletcher GH, 1980. Basic clinical parameters. In Textbook of radiotherapy, 3d ed. (Fletcher GH, ed). Philadelphia: Lea & Febiger, pp. 192–199.

8. Homesley HD, Bundy BN, Sedlis A, Adcock L, 1986. Radiation therapy versus pelvic node resection for carcinoma of the vulva with positive groin nodes. Obstet Gynecol 68:733–740.

9. Komaki RK, Mattingly RF, Hoffman RG, Barber SW, Satre R, Greenberg M, 1983. Irradiation of para-aortic lymph node metastases from carcinoma of the cervix or endometrium. Radiology 147:245–248.

10. Blythe JG, Hodel KA, Wahl TP, Baglan RJ, Lee FA, Zivnuska FR, 1986. Para-aortic node biopsy in cervical and endometrial cancers: Does it affect survival? Am J Obstet Gynecol 155:306–311.

11. Soper JT, Creasman WT, Clarke–Pearson DL, Sullivan DC, Vergadoro F, Johnston WW, 1985. Intraperitoneal chromic phosphate P 32 suspension therapy of malignant peritoneal cytology in endometrial carcinoma. Am J Obstet Gynecol 153:191–196.

12. Bakri YN, Given FT, Peeples WJ, Frazier AB, 1985. Complications from intraperitoneal radioactive phosphorus in ovarian malignancies. Gynecol Oncol 21:294–299.

13. Julian CG, Inalsingh CH, Burnett LS, 1978. Radioactive phosphorus and external radiation as an adjuvant to surgery for ovarian carcinoma. Obstet Gynecol 52:155–160.

14. Klaassen D, Starreveld A, Shelly W, et al., 1985. External beam pelvic radiotherapy plus intraperitoneal radioactive chronic phosphate in early stage ovarian cancer: A toxic combination. A National Cancer Institute of Canada Clinical Trials Group Report. Int J Radiat Oncol Biol Phys 11:1801–1804.

15. Potish RA, Twiggs LB, Adcock LL, Prem KA, 1985. Role of whole abdominal radiation therapy in the management of endometrial cancer; prognostic importance of factors indicating peritoneal metastases. Gynecol Oncol 21:80–86.

16. Potish RA, Abdominal radiotherapy for cancer of the uterine cervix and endometrium. Int J Radiat Oncol Biol Phys, In press.

17. Konski A, Poulter C, Keys H, Rubin P, Beecham J, Doane K, 1988. Absence of prognostic significance, peritoneal dissemination and treatment advantage in endometrial cancer patients with positive peritoneal cytology. Int J Radiat Oncol Biol Phys 14:49–55.

18. Yazigi R, Piver S, Blumenson L, 1983. Malignant peritoneal cytology as prognostic indicator in Stage I endometrial cancer. Obstet Gynecol 62:359–362.

19. Creasman WT, DiSaia PJ, Blessing J, Wilkinson RH, Johnston W, Weed JC, 1981. Prognostic significance of peritoneal cytology in patients with endometrial cancer and preliminary data concerning therapy with intraperitoneal radiopharmaceuticals. Am J Obstet Gynecol 141:921–927.

20. Greer BE, Hamberger AD, 1983. Treatment of intraperitoneal metastaic adenocarcinoma of the endometrium by the whole-abdomen moving-strip technique and pelvic boost irradiation. Gynecol Oncol 16:365–373.

21. Dembo A, 1985. Abdominopelvic radiotherapy in ovarian cancer: A 10-year experience. Cancer 55:2285–2290.

22. Antoinades J, Brady LW, Lewis GC, 1976. The management of Stage III carcinoma of the endometrium. Cancer 38:1838–1842.

23. Bruckman JE, Bloomer WD, Marck A, Ehrmann RL, Knapp RC, 1980. Stage III adenocarcinoma of the endometrium: two prognostic groups. Gynecol Oncol 9:12–17.

24. Hendrickson M, Ross J, Eifel P, Martinez A, Kempson R, 1982. Uterine papillary serous carcinoma: A highly malignant form of endometrial adenocarcinoma. Am J Surg Pathol 6:93–108.

25. Jeffrey JF, Krepart GV, Lotocki RJ, 1986. Papillary serous adenocarcinoma of the endometrium. Obstet Gynecol 67:670–674.

26. Fountain KS, Malkasian GD, 1981. Radioactive colloidal gold in the treatment of endometrial cancer: Mayo Clinic experience, 1952–1976. Cancer 47:2430–2432.

6. Carcinoma of the endometrium and hormonal receptors

PG Satyaswaroop, RJ Zaino, and R Mortel

Introduction

Carcinoma of the endometrium is the most common gynecologic malignancy in the United States, accounting for 38,000 new cases and 3,200 deaths every year [1]. Although surgery and radiation therapy are quite effective and achieve 80–90% cure rates in early stages, most of the fatalities occur in patients with advanced, recurrent, or metastatic disease.

Effective treatment of endometrial carcinoma with progesterone (P) and progestational agents was originally reported by Kelley and Baker [2]. About 35% of patients with metastatic carcinoma of the endometrium responded to progestin therapy in this study. Since then, progestins have been commonly used in the treatment of recurrent or metastatic endometrial adenocarcinoma, and several groups of investigators have observed 20–40% response rates. A similar response rate of about 30% has also been reported with cytotoxic chemotherapy [3]. Unfortunately, no objective, reliable test is currently available for predicting whether hormonal or cytotoxic chemotherapy would be beneficial in a given situation. Therefore, the studies on the sensitivity of endometrial carcioma to steroids and cytotoxic agents and the development of predictive tests for hormonal and chemotherapy have been the focus of attention of several investigators.

Steroid receptors and endometrial carcinoma

The mediation of intracellular, steroid-specific, high affinity receptors in hormonal responses within target cells has been well established [4, 5]. The receptor molecules selectively sequester and retain steroid hormones within the cell. Thus the presence of receptor molecules within the target tissue is one of the pererequisites for steroidal responses. The degree of response to steroid hormones has been positively correlated with the concentration of receptors in several cell culture and experimental animal models. No response to steroid is elicited in cells devoid of specific steroid receptors. Based on this concept, steroid receptor levels are routinely measured, and

E. Surwit and D. Alberts (eds.), ENDOMETRIAL CANCER. Copyright © 1989. Kluwer Academic Publishers, Boston. All rights reserved.

there is general agreement regarding their clinical value in the management of patients with carcinoma of the breast [6]. Breast tumors that are positive for E_2 receptor (ER) and P receptor (PR) are more likely to respond to endocrine therapy, either ablative or additive [7], whereas those tumors lacking receptors are less likely to benefit from hormonal manipulation [8]. Encouraged by these findings, many investigators have attempted to correlate PR concentrations in endometrial carcinoma tissue with its progestin sensitivity and responsiveness to progestin therapy.

There are several reports on the ER and PR concentrations in endometrial carcinoma [9–12]. Although considerable variation is observed in the receptor concentrations in these studies, presumably due to methodologic differences, there is general agreement with respect to the pattern of steroid receptor levels in neoplastic endometrium. Essentially all endometrial carcinomas are positive for ER, whereas PR levels vary with the histologic grade of tumor; the well-differentiated carcinomas contain high PR concentrations, while there are decreased PR levels as tumors appear anaplastic. Notwithstanding the prevailing consensus regarding the relationship between PR concentrations and histologic differentiation of the tumor, the correlation is far from perfect. Several highly differentiated adenocarcinomas with low PR and poorly differentiated tumors with significant PR concentrations have been reported. These discordant findings may be ascribed to the tissue and tumor heterogeneity that is commonly observed in endometrial carcinoma and is described later. The few correlative studies on PR concentration in tumor biopsy specimen from patients and their reponse to progestin treatment, in a limited number of patients, suggested that although a significantly higher response rate is observed in patients with PR-positive tumor, there is a variable response in both PR-positive as well as PR-negative groups [13–14].

Dynamic tests of progestin sensitivity

The lack of a good correlation between receptor levels and the response of endometrial carcinomas to progestin therapy led to the suggestion that dynamic tests may, perhaps, be better indices of progestin therapy [15]. Several dynamic tests that demonstrate the presence of functional PR by monitoring the end effect of P action were attempted. The in vivo approach involved the determination of specific P-responses of endometrial carcinoma before and after administration of progestin to patients. The in vitro methods depend on eliciting P-responses in cultured explants of the tumor tissue maintained in the presence of progestins. The P-responses tested include the induction of progestin-specific enzyme, estradiol dehydrogenase, and glycogen synthesis. It is noteworthy that all these parameters are essentially extensions of normal endometrial responses to the neoplastic tissue.

Hence, there is difficulty in identifying the observed biochemical effect after progestin administration to be a response of the neoplastic cells or a response due to the presence of any normal tissue. We have previously demonstrated that the P-responses cannot be elicited in cultures of endometrial carcinoma tissue, whereas the normal follicular phase endometrial tissue consistently exhibited progestin sensitivity under identical culture conditions [16]. Careful evaluation of the lack of sensitivity of endometrial carcinoma tissue in vitro indicated that PR is unstable and is rapidly degraded in this tissue, whereas significant receptor levels are maintained under identical culture conditions in the normal endometrium. In view of these difficulties, it is doubtful that any of the in vitro dynamic tests could be of clinical use in the management of patients with endometrial carcinoma.

Tissue and tumor heterogeneity

One of the most confounding factors in all studies directed toward the development of predictive tests of progestin sensitivity of endometrial carcinoma is the complication resulting from multiple levels of heterogeneity [17]. Biochemical steroid receptor measurements are routinely performed on endometrial fragments dissected from hysterectomy specimens of patients undergoing surgery for carcinoma of the endometrium. The receptor levels in the specimen assayed may not be entirely attributable to the tumor, since both neoplastic and non-neoplastic tissues are usually found in the same uterus (Figure 1). Normal and hyperplastic endometria contribute variably to the receptor concentrations in the sample. Further, it is unreliable to separate malignant from benign endometrium by gross examination alone. Even a small fragment of normal endometrium in the tumor can significantly affect the receptor status of the specimen used for biochemical assay.

As mentioned earlier, various studies have shown that PR concentrations vary with the histologic grade of the tumor; i.e., well-differentiated tumors generally contain high PR, though the receptor concentrations decrease as the tumor becomes less differentiated. Histologic and histochemical examination of endometrial carcinoma, on the other hand, usually reveal heterogeneity within single tumors. Conventional architectural and cytologic criteria of differentiation generally reveal subpopulations of neoplastic cells with differing degree of differentiation in different portions of the uterine tumor (Figure 1). For example, well-differentiated adenocarcinoma is frequently identified adjacent to foci of moderately and/or poorly differentiated tumors (Figure 2). Under these circumstances, it is practically impossible to ascertain if the biologic behavior of these tumors is related to one or the other of these tumor cell populations. The biochemical determination of steroid receptor concentrations in "tumor" tissues containing heterogeneous cell populations (normal, hyperplastic, and neoplastic cells of different histologic grade) will invariably lead to erroneous interpretation of receptor data,

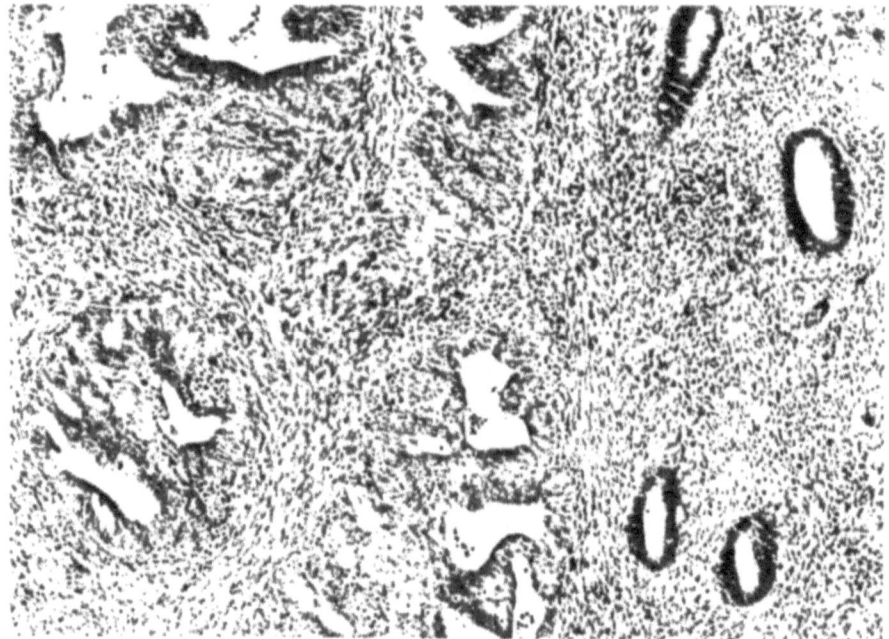

Figure 1. Hematoxylin–eosin stained section of an endometrium containing proliferative phase glands adjacent to well-differentiated adenocarcinoma. (Original magnification: × 25.) Tissue heterogeneity may result from the admixture of normal proliferative endometrial glands (center) with endometrial adenocarcinoma (reprinted with permission from *Cancer* 1983).

as well as of the dynamic tests referred to earlier. Based on these histologic findings, we suggested that development of monoclonal antibodies to the progesterone receptor protein and their use in immunohistologic localization of receptor in tumor sections will help resolve the uncertainty of heterogenous distribution of PR.

Development of the nude mouse model for endometrial carcinoma

The need for the development of an experimental model for the study of the biology of endometrial carcinoma has been felt for a long time. Availability of model systems for human breast carcinoma played a major role in the increased understanding of the mechanism of steroid hormone action and mammary tumor biology. These experimental model systems permit detailed investigations of tumor mitogenesis, which, for obvious reasons, are not possible in humans. Insights into the basic tumor biology, resulting from these studies, played a significant part in designing improved treatment strategies with potential human applications.

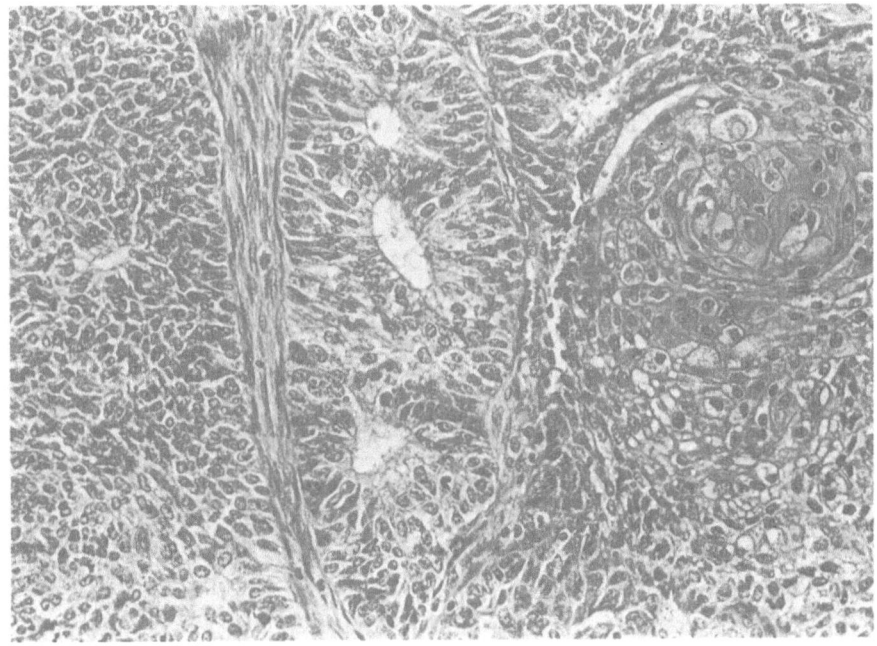

Figure 2. Hematoxylin–eosin stained section of an endometrium with poorly differentiated adenocarcinoma, well-differentiated adenocarcinoma and squamous adenocarcinoma (left to right). (Original magnification: × 100). Tumor heterogeneity is reflected in the intermingling of well-differentiated gland forming portions of a tumor with areas of solid growth or squamous differentiation (reprinted with permission from *Cancer* 1984).

An ideal experimental model for investigating the control of growth of human endometrial carcinoma with steroids and other anticancer agents and for investigating the role of steroid receptors in this process, must fulfill the following criteria:
1. it should be an in vivo system physiologically resembling the human;
2. the tumor under study must be human-derived and must maintain its original histology during the course of the study;
3. tumor growth must be easily measurable;
4. the steroid receptors when originally present should be maintained and modulated;
5. the hormonal milieu must be easily manipulable; and
6. the behavior of the tumor in the experimental system must resemble that observed in humans.

The nude mouse model [18] developed by us for studying human endometrial carcinoma meets the above criteria and thus serves as a valuable tool in deriving various biologically relevant data and in developing rational treatment strategies for this disease.

Scheme 1. Nude mouse model.

Primary endometrial carcinoma
  * Histology
  * ER
  * PR
  * Transplantation into ovexed
    Nude mice (3–5 week old)
      Group 1: Control pellets
      Group 2: E_2 pellets
      Follow tumor growth weekly
      Excise tumor when 1 cm GMD.
Nude mouse tumor
  * Tumor weight
  * Histology
  * ER
  * PR
  * Serial transplantation +/− E_2

E_2 pellets consist of a cholesterol (methyl cellulose) lactose carrier binder coated with E_2 (Innovative Research of America, Rockville, MD). Pellets implanted s.c. maintain blood concentrations of 200–300 pg/ml E_2 for up to 60 days.

The experimental approach used is outlined in Scheme 1. The human endometrial carcinomas were obtained from hysterectomy specimens within 15 minutes of excision. Grossly viable-appearing tumor was collected in chilled nutrient medium and divided for biochemical determination of ER and PR content and for tumor transplantation studies. Randomly chosen pieces from minced tumor specimen were also processed for histologic examination. The histologic grade and the receptor profiles of the primary tumor transplanted into nude mice could thus be compared with the tumor morphology and receptor content after its growht in this experimental system. About 50–100 mg of minced tumor was subcutaneously transplanted in the post-thoracic region three to five-week old ovariectomized, athymic nude mice. At the same time, the animals were subcutaneously implanted with either E_2 or control pellets in the contralateral flank. The steroid impregnated pellets are designed to maintain the indicated blood levels of E_2 for 60 days [19]. The growth of tumors in various groups of animals were measured at weekly intervals using a vernier calipers. When the tumors reached 1–2 cm geometric mean diameter, they were excised and the various parameters listed previously were deterined. The tumors are maintained by repeated serial transplantation in nude mice. A series of human endometrial carcinomas of different histologic grade, steroid receptor content, and growth rates in the nude mouse have been established. The various established tumors and some of their characteristics are shown in Table 1.

Detailed studies have been carried out with some of these tumors in the nude mouse system. These studies have provided insights into the biologic behavior of human endometrial carcinomas and have yielded several impor-

Table 1. Characteristics of human endometrial carcinomas established by serial transplantation in nude mice.

Tumor	Histologic grade	Differential growth with E_2	Passage number	Steroid receptors
EnCa–X	I	+	22	+
EnCa–V	III	–	11	–
EnCa–K	II	–	16	–
EnCa–101	I	+	89	+
EnCa–115	II	+	10	+
EnCa–117	II	+	7	+
EnCa–138	iii	–	9	–
EnCa–139	III	–	5	–
EnCa–143	III	–	7	–
EnCa–144	II	+	10	+
EnCa–154	III	–	6	–

tant experimental tools and biologically and clinically relevant information which are listed below.

1. Biochemical effects of E_2 and progestin in human endometrial carcinoma grown in nude mice [18, 20].
2. Estrogen-like effects of the so-called antiestrogen, tamoxifen (Tam), in human endometrial carcinoma grown in nude mice [18, 21].
2. Morphologic correlates of the observed biochemical responses to E_2, Tam, and progestin in this system [22].
3. Morphologic correlates of the observed biochemical responses to E_2, Tam, and progestin in this system [22].
4. Combination treatment of endometrial carcinoma grown in nude mice with Tam and progestin [23].
5. Characterization of progesterone receptor using E_2 stimulated endometrial carcinoma grown in nude mice [20].
6. Multisite tumor transplantation in the nude mouse to study PR [24].
7. Generation of monoclonal antibodies to human PR [25].
8. Immunolocalization of PR and demonstration of its heterogeneous distribution in primary human endometrial carcinomas [26].

Effect of E_2, Tam and progestin on human endometrial carcinoma grown in nude mice

Investigations on the effects of E_2 on endometrial carcinomas, of varying histologic grade and sex steroid receptor status, grown in nude mice, indicated that E_2 consistently accelerated the growth of the receptor positive tumors, although it had no effect on the rate of growth of receptor negative tumors (Table 1). In addition to its effect on tumor growth, E_2 also augmented PR concentrations in responsive tumors, as might be anticipated in estrogen target tissues.

Table 2. Effect of TAM on tumor weight, ER and PR concentrations in EnCa–X.

| Treatment | Tumor wt (g) | PR concentration fmol/mg of protein | |
		ER	PR
Control (n = 4)	0.82 ± 0.35[a]	263 ± 180	<10
TAM (n = 4)	1.95 ± 0.55	35 ± 26	707 ± 255

Results were obtained from EnCa–X Tumor Transplant 4.
[a] Mean ±S.D. of 4 animals. Reproduced with permission from *Cancer* Res (1984) 44:4006–4010.

The nonsteroidal synthetic compound, Tam, which has been widely shown to be antiestrogenic in breast cancers, exhibited a seemingly paradoxical estrogen-like effect on human endometrial carcinomas grown in nude mice (Table 2). The growth rate of the well-differentiated EnCa 101 tumor in nude mice was increased in the presence of E_2 or Tam (Figure 3), and the response to both these agents paralleled that described previously for the E_2-sensitive, well-differentiated EnCa–X endometrial carcinoma. The increased growth rate was reflected in increased tumor weight, from 0.25 +/−0.05 g in controls to 1.70 +/−1.00 g in E_2-treated and 1.91 +/−0.41 g in Tam-treated animals, and was accompanied by an increase in the cytosolic PR concentrations in the Tam-treated group (Table 2).

Administration of the progestin, medroxyprogesterone acetate (MPA), to animals previously exposed to either E_2 or Tam and whose tumor PR levels were enhanced by this treatment resulted in the characteristic progestin response-increased activity of the enzyme E_2 dehydrogenase. There was no effect of progestin administration on the enzyme activity in the receptor-negative, hormone-insensitive tumors.

Parallel morphologic examination of primary endometrial carcinoma, as well as those derived after growth in nude mice under various hormonal milieu, indicated a high degree of similarity between the original tumor obtained at hysterectomy and, after several serial passages, in athymic mice [22]. Administration of E_2 or Tam to mice bearing the E_2-responsive EnCa–X tumor showed morphologic changes characteristic of these agents in human endometrium. The addition of MPA to E_2 or Tam-treated animals resulted in the appearance of subnuclear and supranuclear cytoplasmic vacuoles, which were intensely stained by Periodic Acid Schiff (PAS). These studies demonstrated that histologic and ultrastructural changes parallel the change in growth and hormone receptor content of tumors in this model system.

Treatment of human endometrial carcinoma in the nude mouse model

The augmentation of PR concentrations in the EnCa–X tumor permitted us to test the premise that combined treatment with Tam and progestin may be

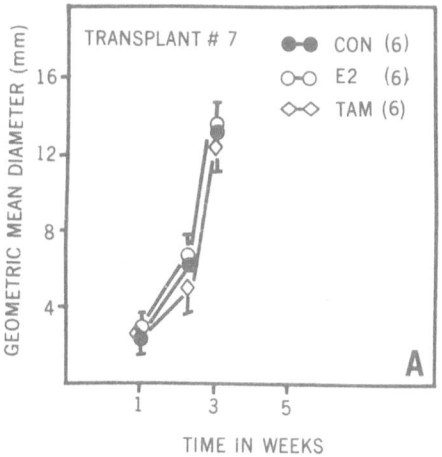

WELL-DIFFERENTIATED ADENOCARCINOMA

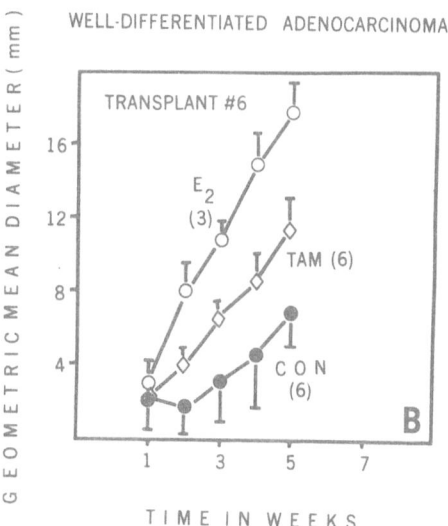

Figure 3. Effect of Tam and E_2 on EnCa–V (A) and EnCa–X (B)tumor growth in nude mice. The number of mice in each group is shown in parentheses. Bars, SD (reprinted with permission from *Cancer Res* 1984 44:4006–4010).

more effective than progestin alone in controlling the growth of this tumor. The prediction was based on several points. As indicated earlier, the presence of PR within tumor tissue is essential for eliciting progestin responses. Since Tam increased PR levels, pretreatment with Tam may be expected to potentiate the degree and duration of response to progestational agents. This postulate was tested in the nude mouse model using the receptor positive EnCa–X and receptor negative EnCa–V tumor [23]. Ovariectomized nude mice bearing either of these tumors were divided into three groups: control, E_2, and Tam. When tumors of a particular group reached about 1 cm geometric mean diameter, they were further divided into subgroups and administered either saline or depo-provera at a dose of 1 mg in 0.1 ml saline, i.m. weekly, and tumor growth rates were determined.

The receptor negative EnCa–V tumor grew rapidly in all three groups, and several animals died before the initiation of progestin treatment. Therefore the effect of various treatments could not be evaluated.

In the steroid receptor-positive EnCa–X tumor, no difference in the rate of tumor growth between saline and progestin-treated subgroups was noted (Figure 4A). The tumors in the E_2-saline treated animals continued to grow rapidly, and all animals were dead by 11 weeks. In contrast, significant suppression of the growth of tumors in the subgroup given E_2 plus progestin were observed for a ten week period, and some of the animals lived up to 20 weeks (Figure 4B). Administration of progestin to Tam-exposed animals resulted in a remarkable regression of the tumor compared to the Tam–saline-treated group (Figure 4C and 5). During the first three weeks of combined Tam-progestin treatment, the EnCa–X tumor continued to grow essentially at the same rate as in the Tam-saline subgroup. This was followed by an arrest of tumor growth for about four weeks, after which there was a decrease in tumor size for the next five weeks. The regression observed on the sequential treatment with Tam followed by progestin was significant, compared to that seen with progestin alone or E_2-progestin treated groups. Subsequently, the tumor growth returned to a rate approximating that in animals treated with Tam-saline. These studies demonstrated that Tam-progestin combination was superior to progestin alone in arresting the growth of receptor-positive endometrial carcinoma and provides the basis for combination treatment of endometrial carcinoma using Tam and progestin in patients with recurrent or metastatic, PR-positive endometrial carcinoma. Sequential, simultaneous, and intermittent treatment modalities with this combination are being carried out in the experimental system, using other endometrial tumors with similar characteristics, to understand the reasons for the resistance phenomenom observed in the above study and to design rational combination treatment strategies for hormone-responsive endometrial carcinoma.

Generation of monoclonal antibodies against human PR

The steroid receptor-positive endometrial tumors (EnCa–X, EnCa–101), when grown in the presence of E_2, contain increased concentrations of PR and thus serve as a continuous source for purifying and characterizing PR. The development of a multisite transplantation system [24] wherein endometrial tumors are grown at four to six subcutaneous sites further increased the amounts of PR-rich tumor. For example, the estrogen-responsive endo-

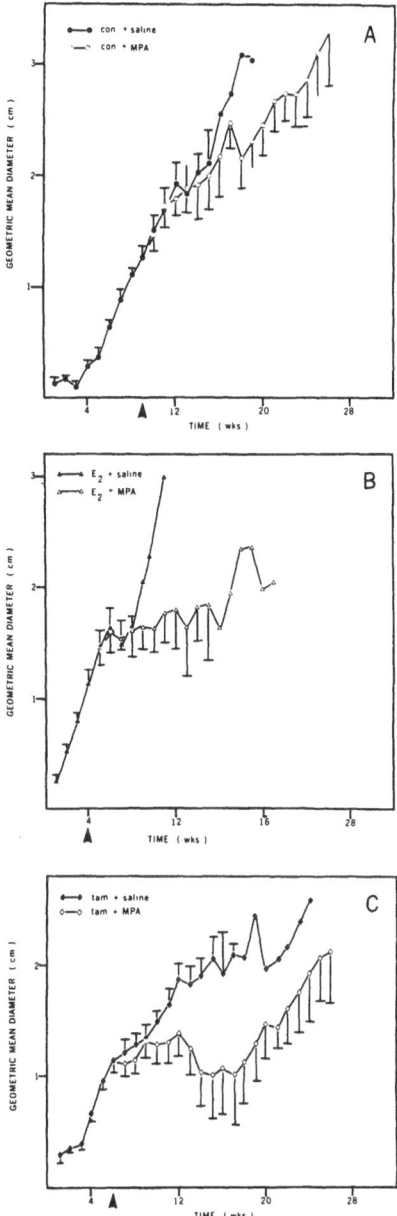

Figure 4. Growth response of EnCa–X to hormonal treatment. Group 1 animals (controls) received no pellet (A); Group 2 animals received E_2 pellets, serum concentration 200–300 pg/ml (B). Group 3 animals received Tam pellets, serum concentration 20–30 ng/ml (C). Tumors reached geometric mean diameter of 1 cm (arrows) in control animals at nine weeks while E_2 treated mice required only four weeks, and Tam-treated mice six weeks. Subsequent additional treatment with MPA resulted in suppression of tumor growth in E_2-treated mice and transient arrest of growth in Tam-treated mice. Bars, SD (reprinted with permission from *Cancer Res.* 1985 45:539–541).

81

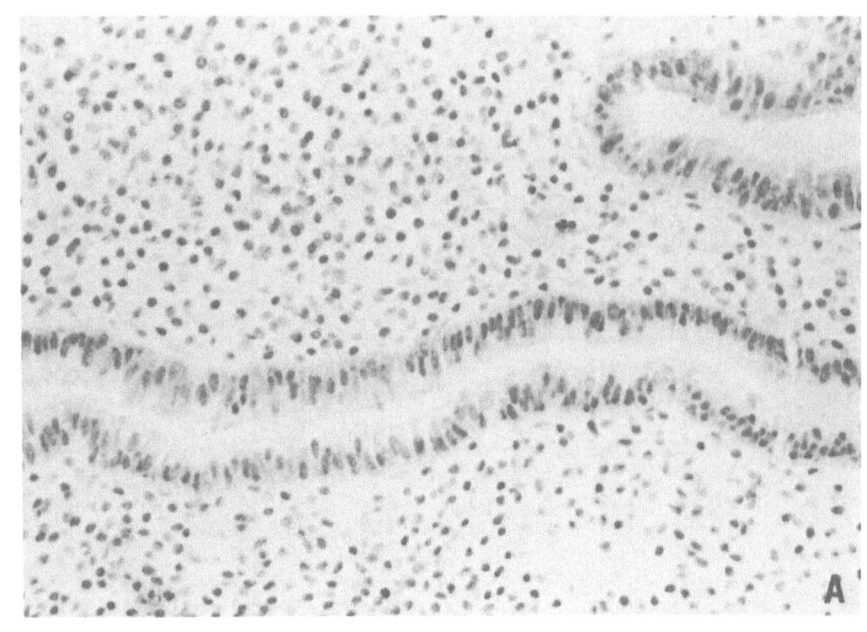

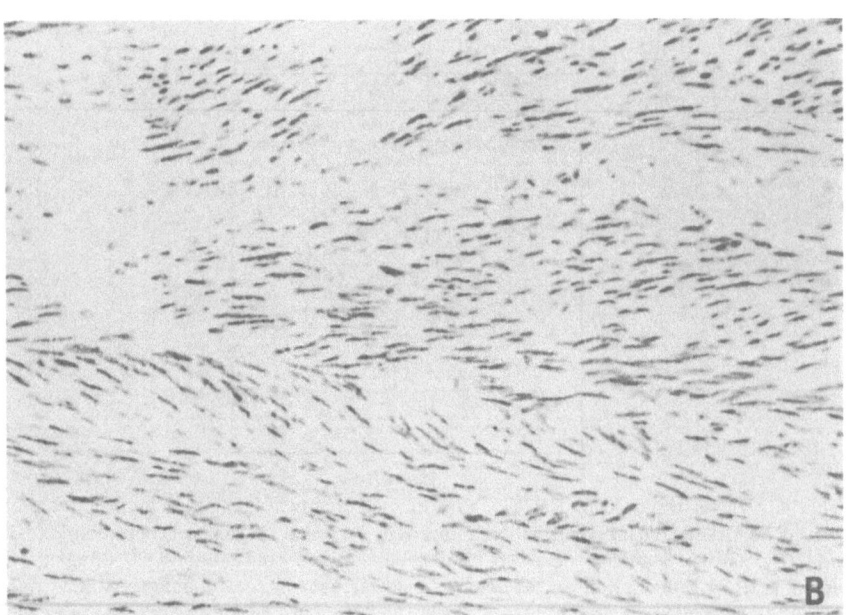

Figure 5. Immunohistochemical localization of PR in human proliferative uterus. There is intense immunostaining for PR in the nuclei of endometrial glands, moderate staining of endometrial stroma (A), and moderate-to-strong staining of myometrial cell nuclei (B).

metrial carcinoma, EnCa–101, grown at four sites per animal in the sustained presence of E_2 in the multisite system, routinely yielded 4 to 5 g of PR-rich tumor per animal in about a four to five week period. This continuous source of PR-rich tumor was utilized for PR purification and antibody generation. Seven monoclonal antibodies, designated hPRa 1–7, were obtained and characterized by immunoprecipitation, sucrose gradient centrifugation, Western blotting analysis, fluorography, and immunohistochemical methods [25]. The immunoglobulin subtypes and other characteristics of these monoclonal antibodies are listed in Table 3.

Immunohisiochemistry was performed on frozen sections of human uterus and showed immunolocalization of PR with each of these seven monoclonal antibodies. The PR localization was confined to the nucleus of target cells. Intensity of immunostaining with each of these antibodies, however, varied as follows: hPRa $7 = 3 > 5 > 6 = 2 > 1 > 4$. The first monoclonal antibody to be obtained, hPRal, was extensively used in PR immunolocalization studies in normal human uteri and in defining the heterogeneous distribution of PR in neoplastic endometrium [26]. Immunostaining was performed for PR in hysterectomy specimens (n = 27) from the various phases of the normal menstrual cycle. Intensity of immunohistochemical reaction was assessed in myometrial, endometrial epithelial cells of the basalis and functionalis portions, and stromal cells. PR localization was confined to the nuclei of target cells and was generally homogenous within the various cell populations. Endothelial cells lining the vasculature were devoid of reaction product. The myometrial cells exhibited moderate (2+) staining throughout the menstrual cycle. Surprisingly, there was very little difference in the intensity of immunostaining between basalis and functionalis layers of the endometrial epithelium. While these cells showed moderate (2+) staining during the early, mid, and late proliferative phases, the immunostaining was weak (1+) during the early secretory phase and negligible during the mid and late secretory phases. The stromal cells displayed essentially similar immunostaining intensity as the epithelial cells, during the proliferative and early secretory phases. However, in contrast to the epithelial cells, the staining intensity was enhanced in the mid secretory phase and further increased during the late secretory phase. While the differential expression of PR in the epithelial and stromal cells during the mid-to-late secretory phases was intriguing, the increased levels of PR in the stromal cells at this stage is consistent with the progestin sensitivity of the stromal cells undergoing differentiation.

Heterogeneity of PR distribution in endometrial carcinoma

Immunolocalization of PR was routinely performed on cryostat sections of human endometrial carcinomas snap frozen in liquid nitrogen. The immunoperoxidase staining was carried out at room temperature using avidin-

Table 3. Summary of the characteristics of hPRa 1–7.

Antibody	Immunoglobulin subtype	Sucrose gradients	Recognition of PR protein blot analysis		Immunohistochemistry
			116,000 mol wt	81,000 mol wt	
hPRa					
1	IgG$_{2b}$	+	+	+	+
2	IgG$_1$	+	+	±	+ + +
3	IgG$_1$	−	+	+	+ + +
4	IgG$_1$	+	+	+	+ + +
5	IgG$_1$	+	+	+	+ + +
6	IgG$_{2b}$	+	+	−	+ + +
7	IgG$_1$	+	+	+	+

Reprinted with permission from *Endocrinology* (1987) 121:1123.

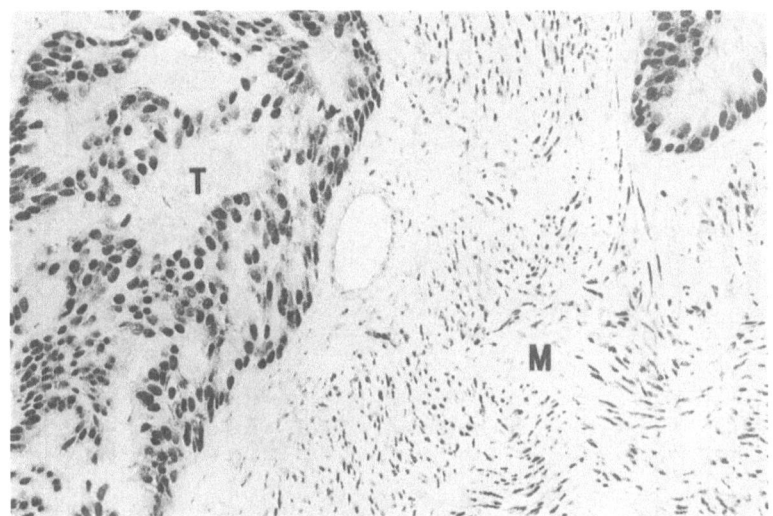

Figure 6. Immunohistochemical detection of PR in human uterus containing endometrial carcinoma. The chromogen is confined to the nuclei of target cells (T) and myometrium (M) but not present in endometrial cells — original magnification X160. (Reprinted with permission from *Cancer Res.* 1988 48:1889.)

biotin complex method, and the intensity of immunohistochemical reaction in individual cells was semiquantitatively graded as negative, trace (tr), weak (1+), moderate (2+), and strong (3+). Immunodetection of PR in human uterus containing endometrial carcinoma again showed nuclear localization in target cells (tumor (T) and myometrial (M) cells), whereas the non-target cells such as endothelial cells were devoid of chromogen deposition (Figure 6).

A comparison of immunolocalization with biochemical determination of PR was carried out in 24 primary endometrial carcinomas of differing histologic grade (Table 4). There was a good correlation between the biochemical and immunohistochemical determination of PR within tumors, the concordance being 83% (20 of 24 cases). In general, the tumors composed of intensely PR staining cells had high PR levels by the biochemical assays, but exceptions were noted. The discordant observations were due to (1) lack of immunohistologic staining for PR in neoplastic cells but low or moderate nuclear staining of adjacent benign tissue or myometrial cells within the tissue section, although the biochemical assay in this tissue was PR positive; (2) immunolocalization of PR in only about 2% of neoplastic cells with a negative PR biochemical assay (Figure 7); and (3) no immunolocalization of PR in neoplastic cell, whereas biochemical assay was positive with 122 fmol/mg protein (Tumor #1029, Table 4).

Of the 24 tumors, 15 were determined to be PR positive by biochemical assay with a range of 122–2,610 fmol/mg protein (Table 4). In 12 of 24 endometrial adenocarcinomas, there was immunolocalization of PR within

Table 4. Comparison of immunohistochemistry for PR with biochemical determination of PR in endometrial carcinomas. Immunohistochemistry for PR.

Tumor No.	Histologic grade	% of tumor stained at each intensity[a]					Intensity of Stain		PR content of biochemical assay (fmol/mg protein)	Correlation[b]
		3+	2+	1+	Tr	Neg	Myometrium	Stroma		
1018	I	30	20	30		20	2+	Tr	2610	+
1025	I		90	10			2+	1+	1654	+
1005	I		20		40	40	1+	Absent	467	+
941	I		30	20		50	1+	Tr	1537	+
1063	I	5	20	15	30	30	2+	1+	916	+
1031	I					100	2+	Absent	1203	−
925	II		90		5	5	2+	1+	433	+
921	II					100	Tr	Neg	c	+
951	II					100	Absent	Absent	c	+
971	II		20	30		50	Absent	Tr	878	+
994	II					100	1+	Absent	c	+
1041	II		80			20	Absent	Tr	364	+
950	II					100	1+	Absent	502	+
891	III					100	Absent	Absent	c	+
893	III					100	Neg	Neg	c	+
903	III					100	1+	Neg	c	+
907	III		20	50	30		1+	Absent	318	+
910	III		100				Absent	Absent	2097	+
995	III			10		90	Absent	Absent	963	+
912	III					100	Absent	Absent	c	+
1028	III					100	Absent	Absent	c	+
1046	III		20			80	Absent	2+	263	+
970	III			2		98	Absent	Absent	c	−
1029	III					100	Tr	Absent	122	−

[a] Intensity of reaction graded as follows: Neg, negative; Tr, trace; 1+, weak; 2+, moderate; 3+, strong.

[b] (+) immunohistochemical staining of tumor for PR and a positive biochemical assay for PR, or (−) absence of staining of tumor for PR and a negative biochemical assay for PR.

[c] <50 fmol/mg protein.

Reprinted with permission from *Cancer Res* (1988) 48:1889.

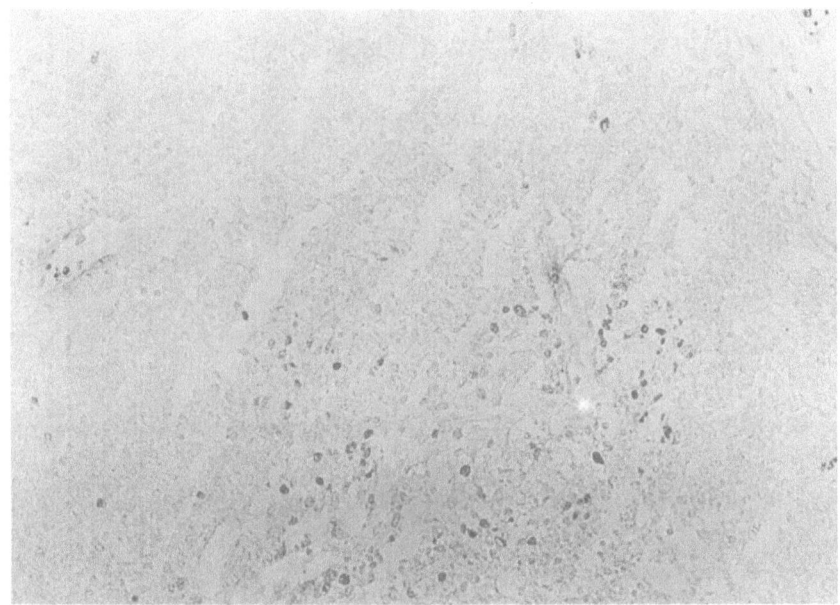

Figure 7. Immunolocalization of PR in about 2% of neoplastic cells from an endometrial carcinoma that was negative by biochemical assay for PR.

the nuclei of neoplastic cells. Immunolocalization of PR was more frequent in the well-differentiated tumors, with the following distribution: Grade 1 — five of six tumors positive; Grade 2 — three of seven tumors positive; Grade 3 — five of 11 tumors positive. The proportion of positive cells and the intensity of the reaction was highly variable within the positive tumors (Table 4). Within individual tissue sections of tumors that appeared relatively uniform by conventional histologic criteria, there was frequently marked heterogeneity in the localization of PR. This variability was observed not only when microscopic fields were compared, but also when adjacent neoplastic glands were compared, and even among the cells comprising an individual neoplastic gland (Figure 8).

The variability in PR content and distribution was also assessed by examination of four noncontiguous sites in each of two uteri containing large endometrial tumors that essentially covered the anterior and posterior lining of the corpus. The tumors were well-differentiated (Grade 1) and appeared uniform by histologic criteria. Binding assays from each of the four sites showed PR concentrations ranging from 829 to 1878 (#941) and 1536 to 2765 (#1018) fmol/mg cytosol protein (Table 5). There was a striking variability at different sites of each tumor in the intensity and proportion of neoplastic cells nuclei that stained for PR. For instance, the proportion of PR immunostaining neoplastic cells ranged from 20% to 90% when two sites in Tumor #941 were compared (Figure 9, A–D). There was also pro-

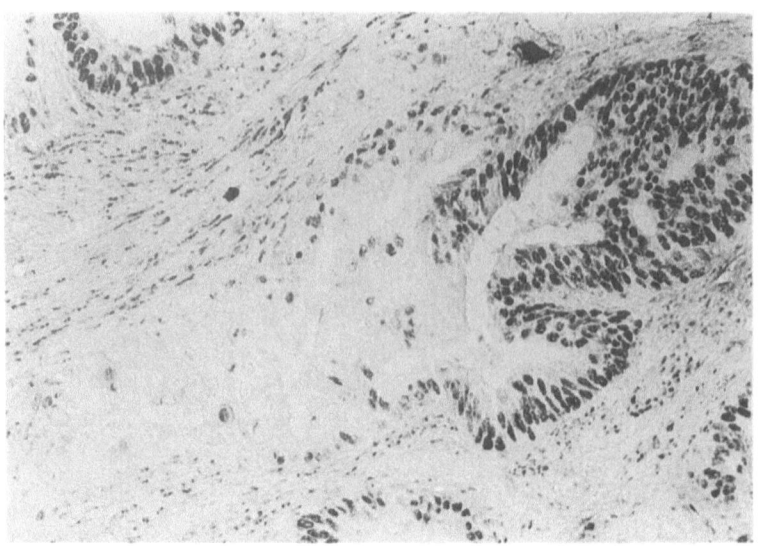

Figure 8. Heterogenous immunostaining for PR within a single neoplastic gland of endometrial adenocarcinoma. Chromogen is present within the neoplastic nuclei on right but is absent from nuclei on left. (Original magnification X160.) NOTE: Positive immunostaining of endometrial stroma surrounding the entire neoplastic gland (reprinted with permission from *Cancer Res.* 1988 48:1889).

nounced staining variability when different microscopic fields from a single site were examined. The immunostaining intensity varied from trace to 2+ among the nuclei of cells comprising individual neoplastic glands. Non-neoplastic endometrial stromal and myometrial cell nuclei surrounding the clusters of tumor cells also displayed PR localization of varying intensity.

The above studies clearly illustrate that PR immunolocalization on tumor sections with monoclonal antibodies provides information not evident from the quantitative biochemical assays of PR. The ability to determine the distribution, proportion, and relative intensity of immunostaining within individual tumors of heterogeneous cells is extremely valuable. Unfortunately, quantitation of immunohistochemical reaction within individual cells is not possible at the present time. Therefore, both biochemical and immunohistochemical assays may have to be performed in studies of endocrine management of patients with endometrial carcinoma. The PR immunolocalization studies described earlier further suggest that failure of some PR-positive endometrial carcinoma patients to respond to progestin therapy might be due to (1) PR-negative tumors falsely disignated as PR-positive, due to contamination by PR-rich non-neoplastic endometrium or myometrium, and (2) failure to respond by PR-negative subpopulations within a tumor containing PR-positive cells. Simultaneous biochemical and immunohistochemical determination of PR in these patients will aid in resolving this issue.

Table 5. Multisite sampling for PR in endometrial carcinoma: Immunohistochemistry for PR.

| Tumor No. | Histologic grade | % of tumor stained at each Intensity[a] | | | | | Intensity of stain | | PR content of biochemical assay (fmol/mg protein) |
		3+	2+	1+	Tr	Neg	Myometrium	Stroma	
941									
A	I		10	20		70	1+	Tr	939
B	I			10	10	80	1+	Tr	829
C	I		50	30	10	10	1+	Tr	1,248
D	I		70	20		10	1+	Tr	1,878
1018									
A	I	5	30	30		35	2+	Tr	1,536
B	I	25	25	45		0	2+	Tr	2,718
C	I	25	25	30		20	2+	Tr	2,765
D	I	15	15	40	10	20	1+	1+	1,696

Four noncontiguous sites removed from each of 2 hysterectomy specimens and immunostained with hPRa–1 as described under 'Materials and Methods.'

[a] Intensity of reaction graded as follows: Neg, negative; Tr, trace; 1+, weak; 2+, moderate; 3+, strong.
Reprinted with permission from *Cancer Res* (1988) 48:1889.

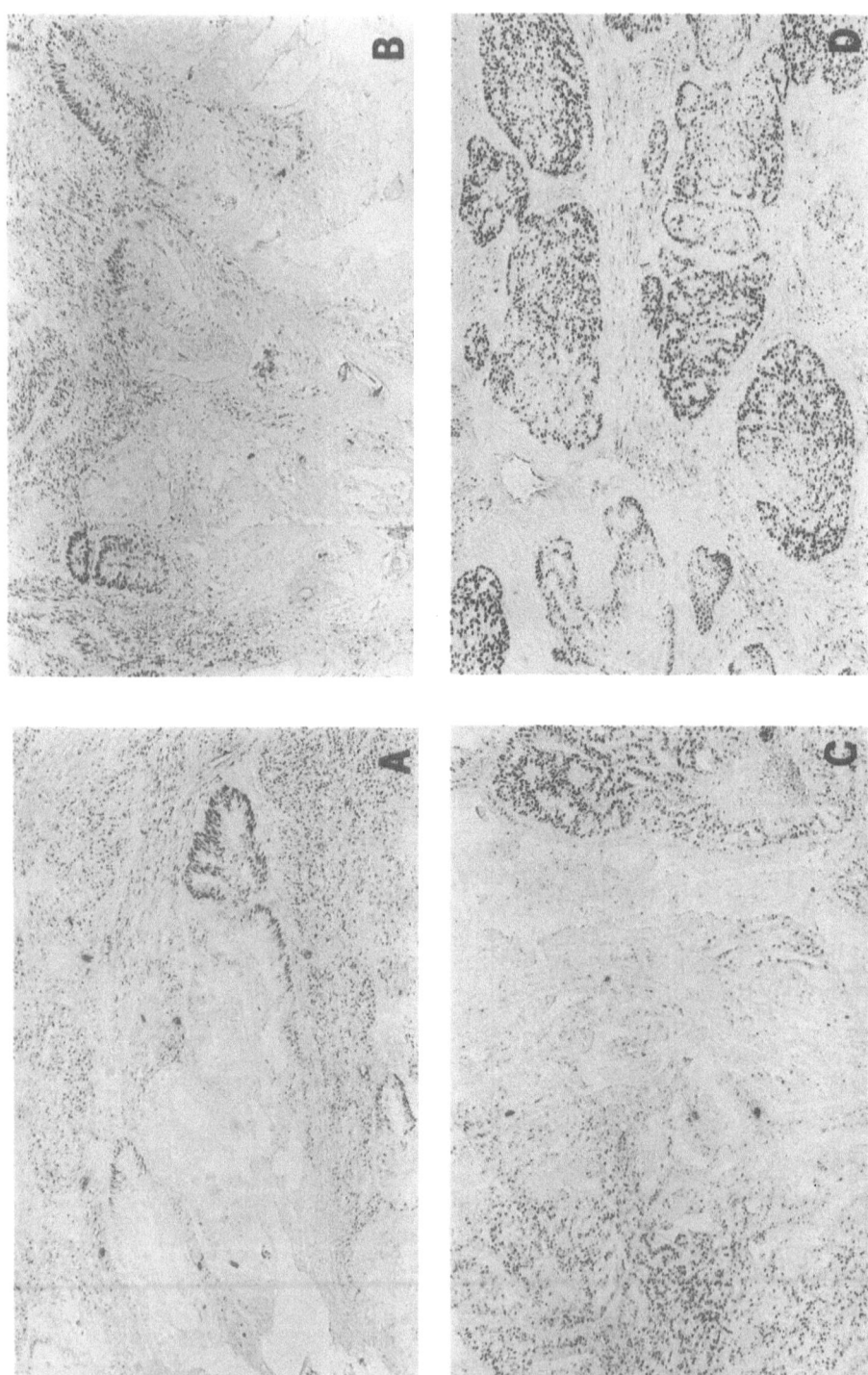

90

References

1. Silverberg E, 1982. Cancer statistics. CA 32:18–42.
2. Kelley RM, Baker WH, 1960. Progestational agents in the treatment of carcinoma of the endometrium. N Engl J Med 264:216–222.
3. Deppe E, 1984. Chemotherapy of endometrial carcinoma. *In* Chemotherapy of Gynecologic Cancer, (Deppe D, ed) New York: Alan R. Liss, pp. 139–150.
4. Jensen EU, DeSombre ER, 1972. Mechanism of action of female sex hormones. Annu Rev Biochem 41:203–230.
5. Gorski J, Ganong F, 1976. Current models of steroid hormone action: A critique. Annu Rev Physiol 38:425–450.
6. McGuire WL, Carbone PO, Vollmer EP, 1975. Estrogen Receptors in Human Breast Cancer. New York: Raven Press.
7. Allegra JC, Lippman ME, Thompson EB, Simon R, Bartock A, Green L, Hupp KK, Do HMI, Aitken SC, Warren R, 1978. Relationship between the progesterone, androgen, and glucocorticoid receptor and response rate to endocrine therapy in metastatic breast cancer. Cancer Treat Rep 62:1281–1286.
8. McGuire WL, 1978. Hormones, Receptors and Breast Cancer. New York: Raven Press.
9. Mortel R, Zaino RJ, Satyaswaroop PG, 1984. Sex steroid receptors and hormonal treatment of endometrial cancer. *In* Chemotherapy of Gynecologic Cancer, (Deppe G, ed). New York: Alan R Liss pp. 125–138.
10. Martin PM, Rolland PH, Gammere M, Serment H, Toga M, 1979. Estradiol and progesterone receptors in normal and neoplastic endometriums: Correlations between receptors, histopathological examinations and clinical responses under progestin therapy. Int J Cancer 24:324–329.
11. Benraad TJ, Friberg LG, Koenders AJM, Kullander S, 1980. Do estrogen and progesterone receptors in metastasizing endometrial cancers predict the response to gestagen therapy? Acta Obstet Gynecol Scand 59:155–159.
12. Creasman WT, McCarty KS,Sr, Barton TK, McCarty KS,Sr, 1980. Clinical correlates of estrogen and progesterone binding proteins in human endometrial adenocarcinoma. Obstet Gynecol 55:363–370.
13. McCarty KS,Jr, Barton TK, Fetter BF, Creasman WT, McCarty KS,Sr, 1979. Correlation of estrogen and progesterone receptors with histologic differentiation in endometrial adenocarcinoma. Am J Pathol 96:171–183.
14. Martin PM, 1982. Endometrial cancer: Correlations between estrogen and progestin receptor status, histopathological findings, and clinical responses during progestin therapy. Excerpta Med Int Can Series 611:333–349.
15. Mortel R, Levy C, Wolff J–P, Nicholas J–C, Robel P, Baulieu E–E, 1981. Female sex steroid receptors in postmenopausal endometrial carcinoma and biochemical response to antiestrogen. Cancer Res 41:1140–1147.
16. Satyaswaroop PG, Mortel R, 1982. Failure of progestins to induce estradiol dehydrogenase activity in endometrial carcinoma. Cancer Res 42:1322–1325.
17. Mortel R, Zaino RJ, Satyaswaroop PG, 1984. Heterogeneity and progesterone receptor distribution in endometrial adenocarcinoma. Cancer 53:113–116.
18. Satyaswaroop PG, Zaino R, Mortel R, 1983. Human endometrial adenocarcinoma transplanted into nude mice: Growth regulation by estradiol. Science 219:58–60.

Figure 9. Heterogeneity in immunolocalization of PR in an endometrial carcinoma (#941) examined at multiple sites. The estimate of percentage of neoplastic cell nuclei containing chromogen varied among the sites. (Original magnification X62.) A — 30% positive (PR assay — 939 fmol/mg protein); B — 20% positive (PR assay — 829 fmol/mg protein); C — 90% positive (PR assay — 1,248 fmol/mg protein); D — 90% positive (PR assay — 1,878 fmol/mg protein). (Reprinted with permission from *Cancer Res.* 1988 48:1889.)

19. Satyaswaroop PG, Zaino RJ, Mortel R, 1987. Steroid receptors and human endometrial carcinoma: Studies in a nude mouse model. Ca Metastas Rev 6:223–241.
20. Clarke CL, Satyaswaroop PG, 1985. Photoaffinity labeling of the progesterone receptor from human endometrial carcinoma. Cancer Res 45:5417–5420.
21. Satyaswaroop PG, Zaino RJ, Mortel R, 1984. Estrogen-like effect of tamoxifen on human endometrial carcinoma transplanted into nude mice. Cancer Res 44:4006–4010.
22. Zaino RJ, Satyaswaroop PG, Mortel R, 1984. Morphology of human uterine cancer in nude mice. Arch Pathol Lab Med 108:571–578.
23. Zaino RJ, Satyaswaroop PG, Mortel R, 1985. Hormonal therapy of human endometrial carcinoma in a nude mouse model. Cancer Res 45:539–541.
24. Mortel R, Satyaswaroop PG, Clarke CL, Zaino R, 1986. Sex steroid receptors in normal and malignant endometrium. Ann Pathol 6:109–114.
25. Clarke CL, Zaino RJ, Feil PD, Miller JV, Steck ME, Ohlsson–Wilhelm BM, Satyaswaroop PG, 1987. Monoclonal antibodies to human progesterone receptor: Characterization by biochemical and immunohistochemical techniques. Endocrinology 121:1123–1132.
26. Zaino RJ, Clarke CL, Mortel R, Satyaswaroop PG, 1988. Heterogeneity of progesterone receptor distribution in human endometrial adenocarcinoma. Cancer Res 48:1889–1895.

Acknowledgements

The Investigations reported here were supported in part by ACS Cevart PDF239 and NCJ grant PO1-CA40011.

7. Systemic therapy with single agents for advanced or recurrent endometrial carcinoma

Tate Thigpen

Introduction

Endometrial carcinoma, now the most common invasive lesion of the female genital tract with over 40,000 cases annually, is regarded as a curable malignancy for several reasons: (1) symptoms in the form of abnormal bleeding occur early in the disease course, (2) the process at diagnosis is usually confined to the corpus of the uterus, (3) a majority of such lesions are well differentiated, and (4) the resultant cure rate from surgery alone is better than 90%. Despite this evidence of success, overall survival figures show that one-third of all patients with endometrial carcinoma recur within five years of diagnosis; most of these die from the malignancy. Until thirteen years ago, no major effort had sought effective systemic therapy for these unfortunate individuals.

In the last thirteen years, a number of drugs have been evaluated in patients with advanced or recurrent endometrial carcinoma. Two hormonal and three cytotoxic agents have shown definite activity, and certain other compounds have evidenced marginal efficacy. This review will look briefly at the activity of these agents when given alone to patients with endometrial carcinoma.

Criteria for therapeutic efficacy

Clinical parameters which are generally accepted as useful, objective measures of therapeutic efficacy include response, duration of response, progression-free interval, and survival. Clear definitions for these parameters are essential if a study is to provide meaningful information with which to judge specific treatment approach. Prior to 1976, trials of systemic therapy for endometrial carcinoma often suffered from a lack of clear definitions for study endpoints [1]. The data to be presented in this review are largely taken from cooperative group studies, particularly those of the Gynecologic Oncology Group (GOG) and the Southwest Oncology Group (SWOG). These trials offer the advantage of having consistent, clear definitions.

E. Surwit and D. Alberts (eds.), ENDOMETRIAL CANCER. Copyright © 1989.
Kluwer Academic Publishers, Boston. All rights reserved.

Response is defined in terms of objective regression of measurable lesions. A *complete response* is generally defined as complete disappearance of all detectable evidence of disease for a specified period of time, usually at least one month. A *partial response* requires that, for each measurable lesion, the product of the greatest lesion diameter and its perpendicular decrease by at least 50% for a minimum of one month. In some trials, this definition is modified to require that the sum of the products from all measurable lesions decrease by at least 50%. *Increasing or progressive disease* is defined as an objective increase in the product from any one lesion of at least 50% (or, in some cases, 25%) or the appearance of any new evidence of disease within one month of study entry. *Stable disease* refers to any patient not meeting the above criteria (less than 50% increase or decrease). Patients having no bidimensionally measurable lesion are considered inevaluable for response.

The other three parameters are defined as the period of time from study entry (or, in the case of duration of response, onset of response) to the occurrence of a specified event or the date of last patient contact. The event in question depends on the parameter under consideration: progression of disease in the case of duration of response or progression-free interval, and death in the case of survival. Patients lost to follow-up are presumed to have incurred the specified event at the date of last contact.

The use of single systemic agents, particular single cytotoxic drugs, in the management of patients with solid tumors such as endometrial carcinoma has, in general, not resulted in significant improvement of progression-free interval or survival. Studies of single agents serve primarily to demonstrate which drugs have the capacity to kill the particualr cancer under study. For studies of single drugs (phase II trials), therefore, the objective response rate (complete plus partial responses) is the critical endpoint. These data are then used in the development of combination regimens that hopefully will begin to impact on the other endpoints. For these reasons, emphasis in this review will be on the response rate.

Hormonal therapy

Endometrial carcinoma is one of several neoplastic lesions known to be responsive to alterations in the hormonal environment. Two alternative approaches to hormonal manipulation have been evaluated in patients with endometrial carcinoma: progestational agents and antiestrogens.

Progestational agents

Progestins were first reported to cause regression of endometrial carcinoma in 1960 [2]. Over the ensuing two decades, a number of different compounds with progestational activity were evaluated as treatment for these lesions.

Table 1. Reported activity for progestational agents in patients with advanced or recurrent endometrial carcinoma.

Progestin	Route	Patients	Response
Earlier trials			
Medroxyprogesterone [3]	IM	151	34%
Megestrol [3]	IM	125	33%
Medrogenstone [4]	IM	56	30%
Recent trials			
Medroxyprogesterone [7]	IM	114	16%
Hydroxyprogesterone [7]			
Medroxyprogesterone [6]	PO	347	17%

Criteria for response varied significantly among these studies. Those trials that used definitions of response similar to those cited previously generally reported response rates of 30 to 34% to parenterally administered progestins in patients with advanced or recurrent disease (Table 1) [3–4]. Although most responses lasted less than one year, long-term survivors were also observed.

Interest more recently has been focused on the use of oral preparations such as megestrol acetate (Megace) or medroxyprogesterone acetate (Provera). That blood levels of progestin similar to those observed with parenteral drug could be achieved with these compounds administered orally was demonstrated by investigators from the GOG [5]. A subsequent clinical trial of oral medorxyprogesterone acetate suggested, however, that the objective response rate with oral progestins was significantly lower than those reported with parenteral preparations (17% versus 30%) [6]. Another recent study using parenteral progestin also noted a lower response rate (16%) and supported the concept that this lower response rate was not necessarily the result of use of an oral preparation [7].

The study of oral medroxyprogesterone acetate conducted by the GOG [6] employed the hormone orally at a dose of 150 mg/day, based on the GOG pilot study showing that blood levels achieved by this approach were identical to those obtained with parenteral medroxyprogesterone 400 mg/week. The response rate of 17% among 347 patients with measurable disease prompted the GOG to conduct a second study, which randomized patients to receive either 200 mg/day or 1,000 mg/day of medroxyprogesterone acetate orally. Although the trial is still ongoing with no comparative data yet available, the overall response rate of 22% among 193 evaluable patients is similar to that achieved in the first study. Compliance has been confirmed in the second study with measurement of progestin blood levels one month after study entry.

Regardless of what the true frequency of response is, it does appear to correlate with both histologic grade of the lesion and status of estrogen and progesterone receptors. Patients with well-differentiated neoplasms respond more frequently to progestins than do those with poorly-differentiated le-

Table 2. Relationship between response to progestational agents and histologic grade [8].

Histologic grade	Response
Well differentiated	52%
Poorly differentiated	16%

Table 3. Relationship between estrogen and progesterone receptor status and response to progestational agents.

	Response	
Study	ER+ PR+	ER− PR−
Creasman [9]	3/5 (60%)	1/8 (12%)
Ehrlich [10]	7/8 (88%)	1/16 (7%)
Benraad [11]	5/6 (83%)	0/5 (0%)
Martin [12]	13/13 (100%)	1/7 (14%)
McCarty [13]	4/5 (80%)	0/8 (0%)
Thigpen [6]	4/10 (40%)	3/25 (12%)
Total	36/47 (77%)	6/69 (9%)

Table 4. Relationship of histologic grade and percentage of patients positive for estrogen and progesterone receptors.

Tumor	Creasman [9]	Ehrlich [10]
Grade 1	83%	84%
Grade 2	58%	55%
Grade 3	31%	22%
Recurrent	36%	23%
Irradiated	—	21%

sions (Table 2) [8]. Those with tumors positive for both estrogen and progesterone receptors appear to respond more frequently than those negative for both receptors (Table 3) [6, 9–13]. Furthermore, there is a correlation between grade and receptor status, in that well-differentiated tumors are more often receptor positive and poorly differentiated lesions more often receptor negative (Table 4) [9–10]. While these data suggest that patients should be selected for progestin therapy on the basis of differentiation and receptor status, reported series to date are small and uncontrolled; hence, no definitive conclusions can as yet be drawn.

It thus appears that progestins have definite activity against endometrial carcinoma. The optimal dose and route of administration remain speculative at the present time. The role of histologic differentiation and receptor status in patient selection for hormonal therapy is similarly not yet clear.

Antiestrogens

The antiestrogen tamoxifen is the only other form of hormonal manipulation which has been evaluated in endometrial carcinoma. An analogue of clo-

Table 5. Reported activity for tamoxifen in patients with advanced or recurrent endometrial carcinoma.

Regimen	Patients	Response
Tamoxifen 20 mg/day [17]	10	3 (30%)
Tamoxifen 60 mg/m2/day [18]	17	9 (53%)
Tamoxifen 20 mg/day [19]	24	0 (0%)
Total	51	12 (24%)

miphene, tamoxifen is believed to exert its effect through two mechanisms: simple blockade of estrogen receptors [14–15] and direct effects on synthesis of DNA and messenger RNA as a result of translocatino of the estrogen receptor-tamoxifen complex into the nucleus of the cell [16].

Tamoxifen is administered orally in daily doses ranging from 20 to 80 mg. The drug is metabolized by the liver and eliminated for the most part via intestinal excretion. Significant adverse effects are uncommon and include: transient thrombocytopenia and leukopenia, menopauselike reactions characterized by flushes and nausea, and a rare severe retinopathy associated with macular edema and loss of visual acuity.

Three series employing tamoxifen in patients with endometrial carcinoma resistant to at least progestational agents have been reported (Table 5). The first of these used a regimen of tamoxifen 20 mg/day in ten patients and noted three responses [17]. The second series used a dose of 60 mg/m2/day in 17 patients with nine observed responses [18]. The third and largest series involved 24 patients treated with 20 mg/day by members of the GOG [19]. There were no responses noted in this last study. None of these reports provided data on receptor status, and no attempt was made to correlated response with histologic grade or site of measurable disease.

In summary, tamoxifen appears to have possible activity in patients with endometrial carcinoma. Further studies are needed to assess the efficacy of the agent in patients not previously treated with systemic agents and to correlate response with such factors as histologic grade, receptor status, and site of metastasis.

Cytotoxic therapy

As of 1976, little information on the activity of cytotoxic drugs against endometrial carcinoma was available. A review of the literature at that time produced evidence of possible activity for three drugs, but these data were collected from multiple broad phase II trials with varying response definitions [1]. Since that time, fifteen drugs have been evaluated. These will be discussed in three groups: those with definite activity, those with marginal evidence of activity, and those with little or no activity.

Table 6. Cytotoxic drugs with definite activity as single agents in patients with advanced or recurrent endometrial carcinoma.

Drug	Regimen	Prior therapy	Pts	Response
Doxorubicin	Collected data [1]	—	18	7 (39%)
	60 mg/m2 IV q3wk [23]	No	43	16 (37%)
	50 mg/m2 IV q3wk [24]	No	21	4 (19%)
Cisplatin	50 mg/m2 IV q3wk [28]	Yes	25	1 (4%)
	50–100 mg/m2 IV q3wk [29]	No	26	11 (42%)
	50 mg/m2 IV q3wk [30]	No	11	4 (36%)
	3 mg/kg IV q3wk [31]	Yes	13	4 (31%)
	50 mg/m2 IV q3wk [32]	No	49	10 (20%)
Carboplatin	400 mg/m2 IV q4wk [36]	No	25	7 (28%)
	400 mg/m2 IV q4wk [37]	No	27	9 (33%)

Active drugs

There are three drugs which have demonstrated definite activity against endometrial carcinoma: doxorubicin, cisplatin, and carboplatin (Table 6).

Doxorubicin. Doxorubicin is an anthracycline antibiotic, the hydroxylated congener of daunorubicin. The drug exerts its effect by intercalation between nucleotide pairs in DNA to prevent DNA-directed RNA and DNA transcription [20]. The drug is active in all phases of the cell cycle; maximally cytotoxic in S phase, it is clearly not phase specific [21].

The drug is usually administered via an intravenous bolus and distributed throughout tissues, except for the central nervous system, over a short period of time with an initial plasma half-life of 30 minutes [22]. Drug excretion occurs primarily through the biliary tract; hence impairment of hepatic function necessitates modification of drug dose. A small amount of the drug is eliminated via the kidneys; hence, the urine can exhibit a red color after drug administration.

Significant adverse effects include myelosuppression, cardiotoxicity, and dermatologic effects (including significant extravasation injury). The acute dose-limiting toxicity is myelosuppression manifested primarily as leukopenia with a nadir between days 10 and 14 after drug administration. Cardiotoxicity limits the cumulative dose of doxorubicin which may be given. Although acute cardiotoxic reactions may be seen, intractable congestiv heart failure becomes increasingly more common as cumulative dose exceeds 500 mg/m2.

Collected data from broad phase II studies prior to 1976 documented seven responses among 18 patients with advanced or recurrent endometrial carcinoma [1]. This suggested activity led to a larger phase II trial by the GOG. Employing a dose of 60 mg/m2 every three weeks, this study yielded 16 responses, eleven complete, among 43 evaluable patients [23]. Median survival for complete responders was 14 months and for partial responders 6.8 months, with an overall median survival of 6.8 months. Confirming this observed activity was a trial of the Eastern Cooperative Oncology Group (ECOG), which used a dose of 50 mg/m2 every three weeks and noted four responses, all partial, among 21 patients [24]. From a subsequent GOG Phase III study, doxorubicin as a control arm at a dose of 60 mg/m2 every three weeks resulted in 29 responses, seven complete, among 130 evaluable patients [25]. The overall median survival of 7.1 months was essentially identical to the earlier GOG study. Toxicity was similar in all three reports.

The Phase II data indicate three important facts: (1) doxorubicin has definite activity against advanced or recurrent endometrial carcinoma; (2) the drug is well tolerated by a patient population that has generally been regarded as at-risk for significant adverse effects because of concomitant diseases and age; and (3) the overall survival impact of single agent therapy in patients with advanced or recurrent disease is minimal.

Cisplatin.   Cisplatin (cis–diamminedichloroplatinum II) is a planar inorganic coordination complex of the heavy metal, platinum. The first of a number of heavy metal compounds to have documented efficacy in cancer therapy, the drug appears to act as a bifunctional alkylating agent with no evidence of cell-cycle specificity [26].

The drug is administered intravenously at rates that have varied from an intravenous bolus to a twenty-four hour infusion. As a single agent, the drug is given at doses ranging from 50 mg/m2 to 120 mg/m2 every three to four weeks. After administration, cisplatin exhibits an initial rapid plasma clearance of one hour or less, followed by a slower secondary phase with a half-life that approximates 60 hours [27]. Extensive protein binding probably accounts for the slower secondary phase. Excretion is primarily via the kidneys.

Adverse effects are numerous. The most significant of these include: nephrotoxicity, neurotoxicity, ototoxicity, allergic reactions, emesis, and, to a lesser extent, myelosuppression. Nephrotoxicity is dose-related, is manifested by renal tubular damage leading to azotemia and electrolyte abnormalities (hypomagnesemia, hypocalcemia, and hypokalemia), and is generally reversible after a peak effect between 10 and 20 days after drug administration. Renal damage may to large degree be prevented by aggressive hydration prior to and following drug administration, to maintain a urine output in excess of 100 ml/hour or by the use of such osmotic diuretics as mannitol in combination with hydration. The concomitant use of other nephrotoxic drugs, such as aminoglycosides, increases the likelihood of nephrotoxicity.

While nephrotoxicity was initially the dose-limiting adverse effect of cisplatin, the reduction in frequency of renal damage as a result of hydration led to the emergence of neurotoxicity as the adverse effect limiting cumulative dose. The observed neurotoxicity included paresthesias, muscle weakness, and ototoxicity, expressed initially as a high-frequency hearing loss. These effects related to the total dose received and were only partially reversible.

There are five reported phase II trials of cisplatin in patients with advanced or recurrent endometrial carcinoma. The first of these, a GOG study of cisplatin 50 mg/m2 administered every three weeks in patients who had received prior chemotherapy, noted only one response among twenty-five patients [28]. Subsequent to the completion of this negative study, three other Phase II trials reported significant activity. Seski and colleagues, using a dose ranging from 50 mg/m2 to 100 mg/m2 every three weeks in patients with no prior chemotherapy, observed eleven responses among 26 patients [29]. Trope, again in patients with no prior chemotherapy, reported four responses among eleven patients receiving a dose of 50 mg/m2 every three weeks [30]. Deppe, in patients who had received prior cytotoxic therapy, noted four responses among 13 patients to a regimen of 3 mg/kg every three weeks [31].

These additional reports, primarily in patients with no prior chemotherapy, prompted the GOG to initiate a phase II trial of 50 mg/m2 every three weeks in patients who had received no prior cytotoxic treatment. Among the 49 evaluatable patients, two complete and eight partial responses were observed [32]. This study confirmed the observations of Seski, Trope, and Deppe and established cisplatin as an active drug in endometrial carcinoma.

Carboplatin. The activity of cisplatin in a variety of malignant lesions spurred activity in the development of analogues in the hope that a compound with less toxicity and equivalent or enhanced efficacy could be identified. The most extensively studied of the analogues is carboplatin. The major clinical difference between this compound and cisplatin is the spectrum of adverse effects. Whereas nonhematologic toxicity, such as nephrotoxicity, neurotoxicity, and emesis, comprises the dominant adverse effects seen with cisplatin, carboplatin actually produces infrequent and relatively mild nonhematologic effects. The dose-limiting toxicity of carboplatin is myelosuppression. Although comparative studies of carboplatin and cisplatin in endometrial carcinoma have not been conducted, randomized trials in ovarian and cervical carcinoma have shown the two agents to be therapeutically equivalent [33–35].

Carboplatin has been tested against endometrial carcinoma in two phase II trials involving patients with advanced or recurrent endometrial carcinoma not previously exposed to chemotherapy. Long and colleagues, in a study of the North Central Cancer Treatment Group (NCCTG), administered 400 mg/m2 intravenously every four weeks to nine patients and 300 mg/m2 to 16 patients [36]. Seven partial responses were observed among the 25 patients. Supporting the conclusion that the drug is active is a recently reported study of the Southwest Oncology Group (SWOG) [37]. This study administered 400 mg/m2 every four weeks to 27 evaluable patients. Three

Table 7: Cytotoxic drugs with marginal activity in patients with advanced or recurrent endometrial carcinoma.

Drug	Regimen	Prior therapy	Response
Hexamethylmelamine	8 mg/kg/day [38]	No	6/20 (30%)
	280 mg/m2 d1–14 q4wk [39]	No	3/34 (9%)
Vinblastine	1.5 mg/m2 CI d1–5 q3wk [40]	Yes	4/34 (12%)
AZQ	30 mg/m2 IV q3wk [41]	Yes	3/27 (11%)
MGBG	500 mg/m2 IV wkly [42]	—	3/21 (14%)

complete and six partial responses were observed. In both of these trials, the median survival was similar to that observed with the single agents doxorubicin and cisplatin. Carboplatin thus is a clearly active drug in the treatment of patients with advanced or recurrent endometrial carcinoma.

Marginally active drugs

Recent reports suggest marginal activity against endometrial carcinoma for four drugs: hexamethylmelamine, vinblastine, aziridinylbenzoquinone, and MGBG (Table 7).

Hexamethylmelamine.   In a small series of 20 patients treated with 8 mg/kg/day of hexamethylmelamine, six responses were observed [38]. This suggestion of activity prompted the GOG to conduct a larger phase II trial of a schedule of 280 mg/m2/day for fourteen days every four weeks in patients with advanced or recurrent disease not previously treated with cytotoxic drugs. Among 34 patients evaluable for response, only three partial responses were observed [39]. The GOG concluded that the drug had, at best, marginal activity; there are no plans for further study of the compound in patients with endometrial carcinoma.

Vinblastine.   The SWOG undertook a phase II study of vinblastine 1.5 mg/m2/day over five days as a continuous infusion [40]. This trial was prompted by observations of potential activity in a clonogenic assay. Among 34 patients who had failed on prior chemotherapy, only four responses were observed. While suggestive of marginal activity, these data were considered to warrant no further investigation of vinblastine in patients with endometrial carcinoma.

Aziridinylbenzoquinone (AZO).   The GOG conducted a phase II trial of AZQ at a dose and schedule of 30 mg/m2 every three weeks in patients with endometrial carcinoma previously treated with alternative chemotherapy [41]. Among 27 patients entered, three responses were observed. The con-

Table 8. Cytotoxic drugs with indeterminate activity in patients with advanced or recurrent endometrial carinoma.

Drug	Regimen	Prior therapy	Response
Methyl–CCNU	150 mg/m2 PO q6wk [43]	—	2/5 (40%)
Cyclophosphamide	Collected data [1]	—	7/33 (21%)
	666 mg/m2 IV q3wk [24]	No	0/19 (0%)
5–Fluorouracil	Collected data [1]	—	10/43 (23%)

clusion was that this marginal activity warranted no further study in endometrial carcinoma.

MGBG. The ECOG studied MGBG (methyl–GAG, methyl–glyoxal–bisguanylhydrazone), 500 mg/m2 given weekly with escalation to 700 mg/m2 weekly in 21 evaluable patients with endometrial carcinoma [42]. Eleven had received prior chemotherapy. Three responses were seen among the 21 patients. This marginal activity was thought to be clinically insignificant.

Drugs with indeterminate activity

Three drugs have exhibited some evidence of activity in selected studies with insufficient data overall to permit definite conclusions to be drawn: the nitrosoureas, cyclophosphamide, and 5–fluorouracil (Table 8).

Nitrosoureas. In an early broad phase II study of the GOG, six patients with endometrial carcinoma were included for treatment with either CCNU 100 mg/m2 orally every six weeks (one patient) or methyl CCNU 150 mg/m2 orally every six weeks (five patients) [43]. Among the five patients receiving methyl CCNU, two partial responses were observed. These data, while suggestive of potential activity, are insufficient to permit definitive conclusions to be drawn. No follow-up study has been conducted.

Cyclophosphamide. Collected data from five separate broad Phase II trials of the early 1970s noted seven responses among 33 patients with endometrial carcinoma on a variety of schedules of cyclophosphamide [1]. This suggestion of activity prompted the ECOG to conduct a phase II trial of cyclophosphamide 666 mg/m2 every three weeks in patients with endometrial carcinoma not previously exposed to chemotherapy [24]. Among 19 patients entered onto trial, no responses were observed. Supporting this observation of no activity are two other studies: (1) a dose intensity analysis that suggests no contribution of cyclophosphamide to treatment with a three-drug combination of cisplatin, doxorubicin, and cyclophosphamide [44], and (2) a GOG randomized phase III trial that showed no difference between doxorubicin alone and the same dose of doxorubicin plus cyclo-

Table 9. Cytotoxic with insignificant activity in patients with advanced or recurrent endometrial carcinoma.

Drug	Regimen	Prior therapy	Response
Piperazinedione	9 mg/m2 IV q3wk [45]	Yes	1/20 (5%)
Etoposide	100 mg/m2 IVd1,3,5 q4wk [46]	Yes	1/29 (3%)
Galactitol	60 mg/m2/wk IV [47]	Yes	1/17 (6%)
Razoxane	2.5 mg/m2/wk IV [48]	Yes	0/24 (0%)
Mitoxantrone	12 mg/m2 IV q3wk [49]	Yes	1/19 (5%)
Aminothiadiazole	125 mg/m2/wk IV [50]	Yes	0/21 (0%)
Methotrexate	40 mg/m2/wk IV [51]	No	2/33 (6%)

phosphamide [25]. Based on these considerations, the probability is that cyclophosphamide has no activity in patients with endometrial arcinoma.

5–Fluorouracil. Collected data from seven broad phase II trials prior to 1976 yielded ten responses among 43 patients with endometrial carcinoma treated with 5–fluorouracil [1]. The dose and schedule of 5–fluorouracil varies significantly among the seven studies. No follow-up study has been conducted. The activity of 5–fluorouracil thus remains indeterminate.

Inactive drugs

Seven additional drugs have been evaluated by the GOG in patients with endometrial carcinoma: piperazinedione [45], etoposide (VP–16) [46], galactitol [47], Razoxane (ICRF–159) [48], mitoxantrone (DHAD) [49], aminothiadiazole (ATD) [50], and methotrexate [51] (Table 9). All except methotrexate were tested in patients who had received prior chemotherapy. None of these agents, including methotrexate, exhibited evidence of significant activity.

Conclusion

A total of two hormonal and seventeen cytotoxic drugs have been evaluated in patients with advanced or recurrent endometrial carcinoma. Four of these agents have definite activity against endometrial carcinoma: progestins, doxorubicin, cisplatin, and carboplatin. Four drugs have marginal activity: hexamethymelamine, vinblastine, AZQ, and MGBG. Four compounds have, based on available data, indeterminate activity: tamoxifen, nitrosoureas, cyclophosphamide, and 5–fluorouracil. Finally, seven drugs exhibited no evidence of significant activity: piperazinedione, etoposide, galactitol, Razoxane, mitoxantrone, aminothiadiazole, and methotrexate.

Even the active drugs studied to date as single agents have offered only temporary benefit to patients with advanced disease. The majority of patients so treated survive less than one year after initiation of therapy.

Ultimately, improved patient outcome will depend on identification of combinations of active drugs that will yield higher objective response rates and, in particular, more complete responses. Two current research directions seek to achieve this ultimate objective: (1) continued phase II trials of new drugs to identify more active agents, and (2) randomized phase III trials involvig combinations of known active drugs, such as doxorubicin plus cisplatin, in comparison to the best single agent, which is doxorubicin at present.

References

1. DeVita VT,Jr, Wasserman T, Young RC, et al., 1976. Perspectives and research in gynecologic oncology. Cancer 38:509–525.
2. Kelley RM, Baker WH, 1960. Progestational agents in the treatment of carcinoma of the endometrium. N Engl J Med 264:216–222.
3. Kohorn E, 1976. Gestagens and endometrial carcinoma. Gynecol Oncol 4:398–411.
4. Bonte J, DeCostu JM, Ide P, et al., 1978. Hormonoprophylaxis andhormonotherapy in the treatment of endometrial adenocarcinoma by means of medroxyprogesterone acetate. Gynecol Oncol 6:60–75.
5. Sall S, DiSaia PJ, Morrow CP, Mortel R, Prem K, Thigpen JT, Creasman WT, 1979. A comparison of medroxyprogesterone serum concentrations by the oral or intramuscular route in patients with persistent or recurrent endometrial carcinoma. Amer J Obstet Gynecol 135:647–650.
6. Thigpen JT. Personal communication.
7. Piver S, Barlow J, Lurain J, et al., 1980. Medroxyprogesterone acetate (Depo-provera) vs hydroxyprogesterone caproate (Delalutin) in women with metastatic endometrial adenocarcinoma. Cancer 45:268–272.
8. Billiet G, DeHertogh R, Bonte J, et al., 1982. Estrogen receptors in human uterine adenocarcinoma: Correlation with tissue differentiation, vaginal karyopycnotic index, and effect of progestogen on anti-estrogen treatment. Gynecol Oncol 14:33.
9. Creasman WT, McCarty K,Sr, Barton T, et al., 1980. Clinical correlates of estrogen and progesterone binding proteins in human endometrial adenocarcinoma. Obstet Gynecol 55:363–370.
10. Ehrlich CE, Young P, Cleary R, 1981. Cytoplasmic progesterone and estradiol receptors in normal, hyperplastic, and carcinomatous endometria: Therapeutic implications. Amer J Obstet Gynecol 141:539–546.
11. Benraad T, Finberg L, Koenders A, et al., 1980. Do estrogen and progesterone receptors in metastasizing endometrial cancers predict the response to gestagen therapy? Acta Obstet Gynecol Scand 59:155–159.
12. Martin P, Rolland P, Ganxamerre M, et al., 1979, Estradiol and progesterone receptors in normal and neoplastic endometrium: Correlation between receptors, histopathologic examinations, and clinical responses under progestin therapy. Int J Cancer 23:321–329.
13. McCarty L,Jr, Barton T, Fetter B, et al., 1979. Correlation of estrogen and progesterone receptors with histologic differentiation in endometrial adenocarcinoma. Amer J Pathol 96:171–182.
14. Jordan VC, 1976. The anti-tumor effect of tamoxifen in the dimethylbenzanthracene-induced rat mammary carcinoma model. In Proceedings of a Symposium on Hormonal Control of Breast Cancer. Alderly Park, Sept 24, pp. 11–17.
15. Hahnel R, Twaddle E, Ratajczak t, 1973. The influence of synthetic antiestrogens on the binding of tritiated estradio-17 beta by cytosols of human uterus and human breast carcinoma. J Steroid Biochem 4:687.

16. Lippman M, Bolan G, Huff K, 1976. The effects of estrogens and antiestrogens on hormone-responsive human breast cancer in long-term tissue culture. Cancer Res 36:4595–4601.
17. Swenerton K, 1980. Treatment of advanced endometrial adenocarcinoma with tamoxifen. Cancer Treat Rep 64:805.
18. Bonte J, Ide P, Billiet G, et al., 1981. Tamoxifen as a possible chemotherapeutic agent in endometrial adenocarcinoma. Gynecol Oncol 11:140.
19. Slavik M, Petty WM, Blessing JA, Creasman WT, Homesley HD, 1984. Phase II clinical study of tamoxifen in advanced endometrial adenocarcinoma: A Gynecologic Oncology Group study. Cancer Treat Rep 68:809–811.
20. DiMarco A, Zunino F, Silvestrini R, Gambarucci C, Gambetto RA, 1971. Interaction of some daunomycin derivatives with deoxyribonucleic acid and their biological activity. Biochem Pharmacol 20:1323–1328.
21. Kim SH, Kim JH, 1972. Lethal effect of adriamycin on Hela cells. Caner Res 32:323–325.
22. Benjamin RS, 1975. Clinical pharmacology of adriamycin (NSC-123127). Cancer Chemother Rep, Part 3, 6:183–185.
23. Thigpen T, Buchsbaum, Mangan C, Blessing JA, 1979. Phase II trial of adriamycin in the treatment of advanced of recurrent endometrial carcinoma. Cancer Treat Rep 63:21–27.
24. Horton J, Bezz C, Arseneau J, et al., 1978. Comparison of adriamycin with cyclophosphamide in patients with advanced endometrial cancer. Cancer Treat Rep 62:159–161.
25. Thigpen JT. Personal communication.
26. Roberts JJ, Pascoe JM, 1872. Cross-linking of complementary strands of DNA in mammalian cells by antitumor platinum compounds. Nature (London) 235:282–284.
27. DeConti RC, Toftness BR, Lange RC, et al., 1973. Clinical and pharmacological studies with cis-diamminedichloroplatinum (II). Cancer Res 33:1310–1315.
28. Thigpen T, Blessing J, Lagasse L, DiSaia P, Homesley H, 1984. Phase II trial of cisplatin as second-line chemotherapy in patients with advanced or recurrent endometrial carcinoma. Amer J Clin Oncol 7:253–256.
29. Seski J, Edwards C, Herson J, et al., 1982. Cisplatin chemotherapy for disseminted endometrial cancer. Obstet Gynecol 59:225–228.
30. Trope C, Grundsell H, Johnson J, et al., 1980. A phase II study of cisplatinum for recurrent corpus cancer. Eur J Cancer 16:1025–1026.
31. Deppe G, Cohen, C, Bruckner H, 1980. Treatment of advanced endometrial adenocarcinoma with cis-dichlorodiammineplatinum (II) after intensive prior therapy. Gynecol Oncol 10:51–54.
32. Thigpen JT. Personal communication.
33. Wiltshaw E, Evans B, Harland S, 1985. Phase III randomized trial cisplatin versus JM8 (carboplatin) in 112 ovarian cancer patients, stages III and IV. Proc Amer Soc Clin Oncol 4:121.
34. Pecorelli S, Bolis G, Vassena L, Epis A, Landoni F, Zanaboni F, Vergadoro F, Favalli G, Gambino A, Marsoni S, Torri W, Jannsen N, Mangioni C, 1988. Randomized comparison of cisplatin (P) and carboplatin (C) in advanced ovarian cancer. Proc Amer Soc Clin Oncol 7:136.
35. McGuire WP, Arseneau J, Blessing J, Given F, Hatch K, Creasman W, DiSaia P, Teng N, 1988. Randomized comparison of carboplation (CP) and iproplatin (IP) in advanced squamous carcinoma of the uterine cervix (SCUC): A Gynecologic Oncology Group (GOG) study. Proc Amer Soc Clin Oncol 7:135.
36. Long HJ, Pfeifle DM, Wieand HS, Krook JE, Edmondson JH, Buckner JC, 1988. Phase II evaluation of carboplatin in advanced endometrial carcinoma. J Natl Cancer Instit 80:276–278.
37. Alberts D. Personal communication.
38. Seski J, Edwards C, Copeland L, et al., 1981. Hexamethylmelamine chemotherapy for disseminated endometrial cancer. Obstet Gynecol 58:361–363.
39. Thigpen JT. Personal communication.

40. Thigpen JT. Personal communication.
41. Slayton R. Personal communication.
42. Salyton R, Faraggi D, 1986. A phase II clinical trial of methyl–glyoxal–bis–guanylhydrazone (MGBG) in advanced endometrial cancer. Proc Amer Soc Clin Oncol 5:119, 1986.
43. Omura G, Shingleton H, Creasman W, Blessing J, Bornow R, 1978. Chemotherapy of gynecologic cancer with nitrosoureas: A randomized trial of CCNU and methyl–CCNU in cancers of the cervix, corpus, vagina, and vulva. Cancer Treat Rep 62:833–835.
44. Levin L, Hryniuk W, 1987. The use of dose intensity (DI) analysis to solve problems in gynecologic oncology. Proc Amer Soc Clin Oncol 6:119.
45. Thigpen T, Blessing J, Homesley H, Petty W, 1986. Phase II trial of piperazinedione in treatment of advanced or recurrent endometrial carcinoma: A Gynecologic Oncology Group study. Amer J Clin Oncol 9:21–23.
46. Slayton R, Blessing J, Delgado G, 1982. Phase II trial of etoposide in the management of advanced or recurrent endometrial carcinoma: A Gynecologic Oncology Group Study. Cancer Treat Rep 66:1669–1671.
47. Stehman F, Blessing J, Delgado G, Louka M, 1983. Phase II evaluation of dianhydrogalactitol in the treatment of advanced endometrial adenocarcinoma: A Gynecologic Oncology Group study. Cancer Treat Rep 67:737–738.
48. Homesley H, Blessing J, Conroy J, Hatch K, DiSaia P, Twiggs L, 1986. ICRF–159 (Razoxane) in patients with advanced adenocarcinoma of the endometrium: A Gynecologic Oncology Group study. Am J Clin Oncol 9:15–17.
49. Muss H, Bundy B, DiSaia P, Ehrlich C, 1987. Mitoxantrone for carcinoma of the endometrium: A phase II trial of the Gynecologic Oncology Group. Cancer Treat Rep 71:217–218.
50. Asbury R. Personal communication.
51. Muss H. Personal communication.

8. Multiagent chemotherapy of endometrial carcinoma

Dean E. Brenner

Introduction

Endometrial carcinoma remains the most common gynecologic malignancy. Since the large majority of cases are discovered early as Stage I lesions, cures are achieved by local means. Advanced disease represents a much more difficult therapeutic problem. While the number of women dying of advanced endometrial adenocarcinoma is substantial (3,500), chemotherapeutic trials have not been extensive. Many women with endometrial carcinoma are elderly, debilitated, or obese. Furthermore, initial treatment with minimally toxic progestins induces responses in approximately 30% of treated patients. Therefore, the number of patients with advanced endometrial carcinoma available for study is small. Well-designed, randomized clinical trials are difficult to complete. Most reported studies of systemic combination chemotherapy are pilot studies of promising combinations of active single agents. Empiric combinations of single active cytotoxic agents, though successful for other pelvic adenocarcinomas, such as ovarian carcinoma, have met with failure for endometrial carcinomas.

In this chapter, I review published multiagent chemotherapy trials for patients with advanced endometrial carcinoma. Identification of a few active single drugs appears to have recently improved our ability to obtain tumor regressions. Unfortunately, this has not translated into improvements in survival of these patients. The small numbers of patients with this disease has limited controlled trials to such an extent that it is uncertain whether multiagent chemotherapy is more efficacious than single agent chemotherapy.

Rationale for multiagent chemotherapy

Skipper et al. [1] first demonstrated a synergistic additive therapy effect of two antineoplastic mechanisms, e.g., an alkylating agent and an antimetabolite. The use of different mechanisms of drug action, such as alkylation and intercalation, combined with overlapping toxicity has led to the successful

E. Surwit and D. Alberts (eds.), ENDOMETRIAL CANCER. Copyright © 1989.
Kluwer Academic Publishers, Boston. All rights reserved.

use of multiagent chemotherapy in a variety of neoplasms: Hodgkins disease, non-Hodgkins lymphomas, Wilms tumors, and acute lymphocytic leukemia in children [2].

Single agents with antitumor activity against endometrial adenocarcinoma include progestational hormones, cyclophosphamide, melphalan, doxorubicin, cisplatin, and 5–fluorouracil. These agents form the basis for combination treatments of endometrial carcinoma.

Combinations of doxorubicin and cyclophosphamide

Since doxorubicin as a single agent has reported response rates of 19–42% [3–5], it is logical to use it as the basis of combination chemotherapy in endometrial carcinoma (Table 1). While activity with cyclophosphamide was less promising, Muggia et al. [6] published the initial combination experience in a small pilot study of patients. A high response rate (five of eight treated patients responded), including three reported complete responses, encouraged further activity with this combination. Seski et al. [7], with the same combination given at different doses, found a lower response rate (31%), no complete responses, and short durations of response (four months), in a retrospective review of 26 treated patients. The doxorubicin-cyclophosphamide combination formed the basis of the multiagent regimen used at Mt. Sinai Hospital [8, 9]. These investigators reported high response rates, acceptible toxicity, and short durations of response with the combination of doxorubicin–cyclophosphamide–5–fluorouracil–megestrol acetate.

Since the doxorubicin–cyclophosphamide data reported were from small numbers of patients, a randomized, prospective trial of doxorubicin-cyclophosphamide–megestrol versus doxorubicin–cyclophosphamide–5–fluorouracil–megestrol was performed by the Eastern Cooperative Oncology Group (ECOG). They reported no difference in response or survival for any of the treatment arms, including a non-randomized treatment arm of 5–fluorouracil, 1–phenylalanine mustard, and megestrol for patients who were not candidates for doxorubicin treatment because of cardiac problems (Table 2). Response rates were between 17% and 27% with survivals of approximately six months. The randomized, multiinstitutional clinical trial did not confirm previous pilot information and suggested that the combination therapies were no better than doxorubicin or cyclophosphamide alone. New agents, alone or in combination, were clearly necessary.

Cisplatin combination chemotherapy

Cisplatin has some reported single-agent activity in endometrial carcinoma (42% response rate) [13, 14], however, this level of activity has not been confirmed by the Gynecologic Oncology Group in previously treated

108

Table 1. Combination of doxorubicin and cyclophosphamide.

Author	Drugs	Evaluatable patients	Response (%)	CR (%)	Median DFI (months) CR	PR	Median survival (months)	Comments
Muggia [6]	Dox Ctx	8	5 (63%)	3 (38%)	10	10,6	—	Multiple sites, poorly diff responded better
Seski [7]	Dox Ctx	26	8 (31%)	0	—	4	—	Retrospective analysis, patients prev treated with progestins
Bruckner [8]	Dox Ctx 5–FU Megestrol	7	6 (86%)	3 (43%)	1–5+		—	Preliminary trial
Deppe [9]	Dox Ctx 5–FU Megestrol	29	15 (52%)	8 (28%)	5.8	8	CR–12.5 PR–9.6	Larger trial of [8]
Horton [10]	Dox Ctx Megestrol vs Dox Ctx 5–FU Megestrol	56 / 58	15 (27%) / 9 (16%)	4 (7%) / 3 (5%)	—	—	All 6	Randomized ECOG trial showing no differences betw combinations

Abbreviations: Dox = doxorubicin, Ctx = cyclophosphamide, 5–FU = 5-fluorouracil, CR = complete response, PR = partial response, DFI = disease free interval, ECOG = Eastern Cooperative Oncology Group.

Table 2. Combinations excluding doxorubicin.

Author	Drugs	Evaluatable patients	Response (%)	CR (%)	Median DFI (months) CR	Median DFI (months) PR	Median survival (months)	Comments
Cohen [11]	L–PAM 5–FU Megestrol	7	7 (100%)	3 (43%)	34–64+	12–20+	—	Early trial
Piver [12]	L–PAM 5–FU Megestrol	11	6 (55%)	2 (18%)	15,4	3.5+	—	
Horton [10]	L–PAM 5–FU Megestrol	12	2 (17%)	1 (8%)	—	—	5.5	Non randomized segment of ECOG study for patients with cardiac disease

Abbreviations: L–PAM = l–phenylalanine mustard, 5–FU = 5–fluorouracil, CR = complete response, PR = partial response, DFI = disease free interval, ECOG = Eastern Cooperative Oncology Group.

patients [15]. Despite these variable data, cisplatin has been added to doxorubicin and/or cyclophosphamide, due to its activity in other female gynecologic tumors, particularly ovarian carcinoma. The results of most of these studies are listed in Table 3. This appears to be an active combination, with response rates between 33% and 56% in the pilot studies listed. Response durations are usually short, and median reported survival rates and usually less than a year. The recently reported randomized study of Edmonson et al. [21] does not support the rest of the pilot data. Responses were low in both the cisplatin-alone arm and the combination arm. Survivals were no different. This randomized study is of importance because of its comparison of single-agent to multiagent chemotherapy. Despite the crossover design for cisplatin-alone failures, there does not appear to be any difference in response or survival between those patients treated with single agents and those treated with combination chemotherapy.

The recently reported SWOG study of Alberts et al. [22] is of interest because it is a pilot trial based upon results in the human tumor colony stem cell assay of Hamburger and Salmon [23]. Response rates, duration of response, and survivals were consistent with other reports for the cisplatin–doxorubicin combination studies. The clonogenic assay was not considered predictive for drug activity for endometrial carcinoma.

Pilot data versus randomized trials

How does one explain the descrepancies between the pilot data and the randomized trials? Many factors are likely to be involved. As with ovarian carcinoma, advanced endometrial carcinoma encompasses a wide variety of tumor burdens, from a small amount of tumor recurring in the pelvis to widespread dissemination in the abdominal and thoracic cavities. Edmonson et al. [21] point out that clinical complete responses, as in ovarian carcinoma, may not be pathologic complete responses, since endometrial carcinoma commonly recurs intra-abdominally. Abdominal responses are difficult to measure due to lack of sensitivity of abdominal imaging techniques. The anatomic location of disease does not correlate to prognosis or response to chemotherapy [6, 10, 19, 21]. Some studies have suggested that grade of tumor predicts for chemotherapy response [6], but this has not been substantiated [10, 19, 21]. Pretreatment performance status appears to correlate to response and survival [10, 19]. Problems with such correlations are likely, due to the small numbers of patients in most of the studies. When a combination is evaluated in larger sample size, possible prognostic and response differences are not confirmed.

For endometrial carcinoma, unlike ovarian carcinoma, resistance to chemotherapy is common at first treatment. Since most endometrial carcinoma patients are diagnosed and cured with local disease, those patients who recur or who present with advanced disease may have a cell population

111

Table 3. Combinations including doxorubicin and cisplatin.

Author	Drugs	Evaluatable patients	Response (%)	CR (%)	Median DFI (months) CR	Median DFI (months) PR	Median survival (months)	Comments
Seltzer [16]	Dox DDP	9	3 (33%)	1 (11%)	12	3,8+	—	75% of patients being treated primarily responded
Trope [17]	Dox DDP	19	12 (63%)	2 (11%)	16+,23	3–19+	11	No prior chemotx, both CRs vaginal disease only
Pasmantier [18]	Dox DDP	16	13 (81%)	6 (38%)	—	—	10	2/6 CRs on lap had persistant disease; poorer survival in prev treated patients
Turbow [19]	Dox DDP Ctx	19	7 (37%)	2 (11%)	3	8	10	
Hancock [20]	Dox DDP	18	10 (56%)	5 (28%)	—	—	—	All patients prev treated, most with hormones
Edmonson [21]	DDP vs DDP Dox Ctx	14 16	3 (21%) 5 (24%)	1 (7%) 0	— —	— —	4.2 6.7	Randomized, stratified; DDP alone failures Rx with Dox+Ctx
Alberts [22]	Dox	44	13	3	All — 8	—	10	Pilot study based upon clonogenic assay

Abbreviations: Dox = doxorubicin, Ctx = cyclophosphamide, DDP = cisplatin, CR = complete response, PR = partial response, DFI = disease free interval, Chemotx = chemotherapy.

more resistant to systemic therapy than those patients presenting with local disease.

Dose intensity analysis

Levin and Hryniuk [24] have recently suggested that dose intensity analysis may clarify the contributions of antineoplastic agents to a combination chemotherapy regimen. Their dose intensity analysis methodology [25] defines the amount of drug given per unit time, expressed as $mg/m^2/wk$ regardless of the schedule used. The calculation of dose intensity gives equal importance to time delays and dose reductions. It is based on the assumption that scheduling does not directly determine tumor cell kill. For purposes of calculating dose intensity, it does not matter if chemotherapy is given monthly, five days a month, or three times a month. For all schedules, the amount of drug delivered per unit time is converted to the standard form $mg/m^2/wk$. It is then possible to compare regimens by arbitrarily designating one regimen as the standard, expressing every regimen relative to that standard, and correlating the outcome by comparing response rate to average dose intensity.

In Figures 1A and 1B, the dose intensity analysis for endometrial carcinoma regimens suggests that cyclophosphamide does not contribute to treatment efficacy. The analysis in Figure 1A is nonlinear and the points represent dose intensity, including cyclophosphamide, in the calculation. When cyclophosphamide is removed from the dose intensity calculation, as shown in Figure 1B, a linear correlation between complete and partial response rate and average dose intensity exists. This work suggests that one method of improving response rate is to increase the doses of doxorubicin and cisplatin and to eliminate cyclophosphamide from the treatment regimens.

Dose intensity calculations may be helpful for the formulation of new prospective trials of combination chemotherapy regimens. Since this methodology is a retrospective analysis of published data, care should be exercised before basing treatment decisions on data derived by this analysis. Prospective validation of this methodology is underway but is incomplete and not being performed for endometrial carcinoma.

Summary and conclusions

Minimal experience in the use of combination chemotherapy for endometrial carcinoma is published. This is due to the small numbers of patients who receive systemic cytotoxic chemotherapy because of age, physical status, and prior treatment with hormones. Published studies of combination chemotherapy are based primarily on doxorubicin–cisplatin–

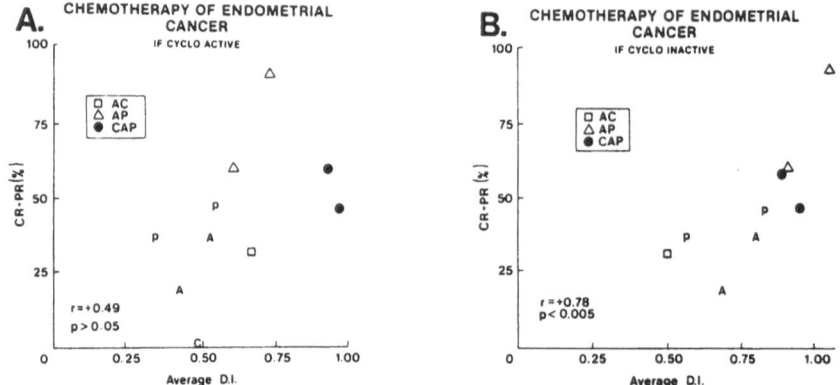

Figure 1. Clinical response of endometrial cancer versus average relative dose intensity of chemotherapy: A. calculations with cyclophosphamide; B. calculations without cyclophosphamide in which the correlation is significant. (Reprinted with permission from Levin, L, Hryniuk W, 1987. The application of dose intensity to problems in chemotherapy of ovarian and endometrial cancer. Semin Oncol 14:12–19.)

cyclophosphamide combinations. While the pilot studies suggest high complete plus partial response rates, these do not appear to translate into improved survival. Furthermore, prospective randomized studies or multi-institutional trials of these regimens fail to show any advantage of multiagent regimens over the studies of single agents. Retrospective dose intensity analysis has suggested cisplatin and doxorubicin to be the two active agents for this disease.

Future directions

New approaches for treatment of this resistant disease may take many directions. Intensive dosing with doxorubicin and cisplatin may be of interest because of evidence from the human tumor stem cell assay and dose intensity analysis that these two agents are probably the most active for endometrial carcinoma. New concepts in resistance reversal may be useful for endometrial carcinoma. If resistant endometrial carcinomas express the multidrug resistance phenotype [27], it may be possible to improve responses to cytotoxic chemotherapy by the addition of reversal agents [28, 29]. New monoclonal antibody drug carriers may be able to exploit hormone receptors on endometrial carcinoma cell surfaces. New bioactive agents, such as tumor necrosis factor, the interleukins, and interferons, are now entering clinical trials. They may provide new therapeutic tools to use in combination with other standard agents to treat this resistant disease.

References

1. Skipper HC, Chapman JB, Bell M, 1952. The anti-leukemic action of combinations of certain known anti-leukemia agents. Cancer Res 11:109–114.
2. Johnson RK, Goldin A, 1975. The clinical impact of screening and other experimental tumor studies. Cancer Treat Rev 2:1.
3. Donovan JF, 1974. Non-hormonal chemotherapy of advanced endometrial adenocarcinoma: A review. Cancer 34:1587–1592.
4. Thigpen JT, Buchsbaum, HJ, Mangan C, Blessing JA, 1979. A phase II trial of adriamycin in the treatment of advanced or recurrent endometrial carcinoma. A Gynecologic Oncology Group Study. Cancer Treat Rep 63:21–27.
5. Horton J, Begg CB, Arsenau J, et al., 1978. Comparison of adriamycin with cyclophosphamide in patients with endometrial carcinoma. Cancer Treat Rep 62:159–161.
6. Muggia FM, Chia G, Reed LJ, Romney SL, 1977. Doxorubicin-cyclophosphamide: Effective chemotherapy for advanced endometrial adenocarcinoma. Am J Obstet Gynecol 128:314–319.
7. Seski JC, Edwards CL, Gershenson DM, Copeland LJ, 1981. Doxorubicin and cyclophosphamide chemotherapy for disseminated endometrial cancer. Obstet Gynecol 58:88–91.
8. Bruckner HW, Deppe G, 1977. Combination chemotherapy of advanced endometrial adenocarcinoma with adriamycin, cyclophosphamide, 5–fluorouracil, and medroxyprogesterone acetate. Obstet Gynecol 50:10s–12s.
9. Deppe G, Jacobs AJ, Bruckner H, Cohen CJ, 1981. Chemotherapy of advanced and recurrent endometrial carcinoma with cyclophosphamide, doxorubicin, 5–fluorouracil, and megestrol acetate. Am J Obstet Gynecol 140:313–316.
10. Horton J, Elson P, Gordon P, Hahn R, Creech R, 1982. Combination chemotherapy for advanced endometrial cancer. Cancer 49:2441–2445.
11. Cohen CJ, Deppe G, Bruckner HW, 1977. Treatment of advanced adenocarcinoma of the endometrium with melphalan, 5–fluorouracil, and medroxyprogesterone. Obstet Gyencol 50:415–417.
12. Piver MS, Lele S, Barlow JJ, 1980. Melphalan, 5–fluorouracil, and medroxyprogesterone acetate in metastatic or recurrent endometrial carcinoma. Obstet Gynecol 56:370–372.
13. Trope C, Grundsell H, Johnsson JE, Cavallin–Stahl E, 1980. A phase II study of cisplatinum for recurrent corpus cancer. Eur J Cancer 16:1025–1028.
14. Seski JC, Edwards CL, Herson J, et al., 1982. Cisplatin chemotherapy for disseminated endometrial cancer. Obstet Gynecol 59:225–228.
15. Thigpen JT, Blessing JA, Lagasse LD, et al., 1984. Phase II trial of cisplatin as second-line chemotherapy in patients with advanced or recurrent endometrial carcinoma. Am J Clin Oncol 7:253–256.
16. Seltzer V, Vogl SE, Kaplan BH, 1984. Adriamycin and cis-diamminedichloroplatinum in the treatment of metastatic endometrial adenocarcinoma. Gynecol Oncol 19:308–313.
17. Trope C, Johnsson JE, Simonsen E, et al., 1984. Treatment of recurrent endometrial adenocarcinoma with a combination of doxorubicin and cisplatin. Am J Obstet Gynecol 149:379–381.
18. Pasmantier MW, Coleman M, Silver RT, et al., 1985. Treatment of advanced endometrial carcinoma with doxorubicin and cisplatin: Effects on both untreated and previously treated patients. Cancer Treat Rep 69:539–542.
19. Turbow MM, Ballon SC, Sikic BI, Koretz MM, 1985. Cisplatin, doxorubicin, and cyclophosphamide chemotherapy for advanced endometrial carcinoma. Cancer Treat Rep 69: 465–467.
20. Hancock KC, Freedman RS, Edwards CL, Rutledge FN, 1986. Use of cisplatin, doxorubicin, and cyclophosphamide to treat advanced and recurrent adenocarcinoma of the endometrium. Cancer Treat Rep 70:789–791.

21. Edmonson JH, Krook JE, Hilton JF, et al., 1987. Randomized phase II studies of cisplatin and a combination of cyclophosphamide-doxorubicin-cisplatin (CAP) in patients with progestin-refractory advanced endometrial carcinoma. Gynecol Oncol 28:20–24.
22. Alberts DS, Mason NL, O'Toole RV, et al., 1987. Doxorubicin-cisplatin-vinblastine combination chemotherapy of advanced endometrial carcinoma: A Southwest Oncology Group study. Gynecol Oncol 26:193–201.
23. Hamburger AW, Salmon SE, 1977. Primary bioassay of human tumor stem cells. Science 197:461–463.
24. Levin L, Hryniuk W, 1987. The application of dose intensity to problems in chemotherapy of ovarian and endometrial cancer. Semin Oncol 14:(Supple 4)12–19.
25. Hryniuk W, 1987. The impact of dose intensity on the design of clinical trials. Semin Oncol 14:65–74.
26. Tannock IF, Boyd NF, DeBoer G, et al., 1988. A randomized trial of two dose levels of cyclophosphamide, methotrexate, and fluorouracil chemotherapy for patients with metastatic breast cancer. J Clin Oncol 6:1377–1387.
27. Moscow JA, Cowan KH, 1988. Multidrug resistance. JNCI 80:14–19.
28. Miller RL, Bukowski RM, Budd GT, et al., 1988. Clinical modulation of doxorubicin resistance by the calmodulin-inhibitor, trifluoperazine: A phase I/II trial. J Clin Oncol 6:880–888.
29. Ozols RF, Cunnion RE, Klecker RW, et al., 1987. Verapamil and adriamycin in the treatment of drug-resistant ovarian cancer patients. J Clin Oncol 5:641–647.

9. In vitro sensitivity of human endometrial cancer to cytotoxic and biologic agents

Charles E. Welander, Charles M. Jones, III, David S. Alberts, and Sydney E. Salmon

Introduction

A goal of cancer research continues to be a better understanding of tumor cell growth and possible ways to modify it. If we learn from preclinical studies which factors are able to modify cell growth, there are oftentimes therapeutic decisions that can be made that ultimately improve patient care. In a clinical setting, the simplest observation to be made is the geographic extent of tumor growth, an assessment made when a patient first presents with a malignancy. Extent of disease determinations have been standardized as tumor stage [1]. Sophisticated imaging techniques and even surgical exploration have been applied as a means to detect clinically inapparent tumor extension. In the example of endometrial cancer, more detailed predictive information following surgery can be obtained by microscopic studies of tumor invasion into the myometrium, the architectural grade (FIGO) and the nuclear grade of the tumor [2, 3]. Predictions of recurrence probabilities can be made, based upon these morphologic and/or geographic parameters. The proliferative activity of a tumor, as determined by flow cytometry, is also significantly related to prognosis [4]. Other biologic parameters that relate to growth of endometrial cancers have been identified, such as the presence or absence of steroid hormone receptors on tumor cells. Receptors can predict tumor growth in response to certain types of treatment [5].

One further in vitro means to evaluate tumor growth is tissue culture of endometrial cancers. Application of colony-forming assay techniques has demonstrated in vitro cloning efficiency of endometrial cancers and sensitivity patterns to various drugs [6]. Both conventional and investigational drugs can be screened in vitro for antiproliferative activity. In vitro 'Phase II Trials' for endometrial cancers are feasible, using such colony-forming assays [7]. Patterns of drug sensitivity of endometrial cancers can be determined, by testing either single agents or combinations of drugs in vitro. When tumor cells are cultured with biologic response modifiers, direct cytotoxic effects of the particular agent on the tumor cells will be noted. If 'feeder cells,' such as macrophages, are also added to the culture, then both direct and indirect antiproliferative effects mediated through the feeder cell population will be observed [8].

In this chapter, data are presented from colony-forming assays of an established cell line derived from a human endometrial cancer and tested with a variety of chemotherapeutic agents. In addition, a large series of primary endometrial carcinomas have also been tested in vitro, using standard and investigational agents. In vitro results of biologic response modifier effects on tumor cell growth are also presented. Finally, conclusions are drawn concerning potential application of these in vitro data to patient treatment situations.

In vitro growth of endometrial cancers

The in vitro studies reported here have been done at Bowman Gray School of Medicine of Wake Forest University and also at the University of Arizona in Tucson. Colony-forming assays have been commonly used to study solid human tumor specimens in vitro since the classic work of Hamburger and Salmon was published in 1977 [9]. Modifications of the technique have been introduced over the past decade and have been described in detail elsewhere [10]. In summary, tumor material representing either primary tumor or metastatic disease in patients with endometrial cancers was obtained from surgery or curettage specimens. Efforts were always made to minimize the time elapsed between removal of the tumor tissue from the patient and processing of it in the laboratory. Tumor specimens were mechanically minced and fragments enzymatically disaggregated by a hypotonic solution containing collagenase. The suspension was then layered over a Ficoll–Paque® gradient to separate viable tumor cells from non-viable cellular debris. The resulting gradient interface contained the tumor cells, which were resuspended in culture medium. Cells were passed through a filter to remove clusters and clumps of cells. At this point, a single cell suspension had been prepared which could either be incubated directly with predetermined drug concentrations for a short period of time or directly mixed into molten agarose and plated in culture dishes. The standard colony-forming assay was prepared with a nutrient agarose underlayer, over which the tumor cell plating layer was added. Individual tumor cells could then form colonies within the agarose matrix. An automated image analysis system (FAS–II, Bausch and Lomb) was used to count tumor cell colonies after they had reached a minimum size of at least 50 micrometers.

Exposure of tumor cells to the various drugs was done either as a one hour incubation prior to plating cells in agarose or by adding appropriate concentrations of drug to the culture dishes after the cells were plated. This method resulted in continuous cell exposure to the drugs for as long as the drug remained active at 37 degrees in a medium containing fetal calf serum.

Occasionally patients with advanced endometrial cancers presented with malignant effusions that contained tumor cells. These usually required very little disaggregation prior to separating out tumor cells for culture purposes. These specimens were then processed in a similar manner to the processing of solid tumors. Established cell lines, likewise, required minimal disaggregation and could be plated in the same fashion. The indirect effect of antiproliferative agents on tumor cells can be studied in colony-forming assays if 'feeder cells' are added. One method has been to add adherent peritoneal cells (greater than 90% macrophages) to the nutrient underlayer. As an example, these feeder cells can be stimulated by interferon gamma to produce a soluble substance that significantly decreases tumor cell growth [8]. Experiments testing biologic response modifiers often are designed with or without feeder cells in order to note both direct and indirect effects of the substance on tumor colony formation.

Drug sensitivity tests on an endometrial cancer cell line

Established cell line HEC–1A was originally derived from a human endometrial cancer, first published in 1972 [11]. It has been continuously passaged in vitro since that time. It is unclear whether this cell line continues to be a representative sample of human endometrial cancers in terms of its drug sensitivity. However, use of established cell lines makes it possible to repeat experiments many times for comparative purposes. Primary surgical specimens from an individual patient rarely allow repeated studies to be done. Figures 1–3 show dose response curves of cell line HEC–1A tested with several commonly used chemotherapeutic agents. The activities of cisplatin and 5–fluorouracil are shown in Figure 1, each demonstrating a dose response curve when tested with the continuous drug exposure method. It is possible to reduce tumor colony growth by at least two logs, using drug concentrations ≥ 1 mcg/ml. In Figure 2, data are shown of HEC–1A cells tested with doxorubicin and cyclophosphamide (4–hydroperoxcyclophosphamide). Using the continuous drug exposure method, parallel cultures with and without macrophage feeder cells were compared, noting that response to cytotoxic drug therapy is not changed by the presence or absence of macrophages. It is again possible with these drugs to inhibit tumor colony formation by at least two logs, compared to control cultures. Data showing the activity of two biologic response modifiers, interferon alpha and interferon gamma, are plotted together in Figure 3. While these interferons have shown some direct antiproliferative effect on tumor cells from other human solid tumors, there was no significant antiproliferative activity observed with HEC–1A cells, whether feeder cells were used or not, up to concentrations of 10,000 units interferon [8, 10].

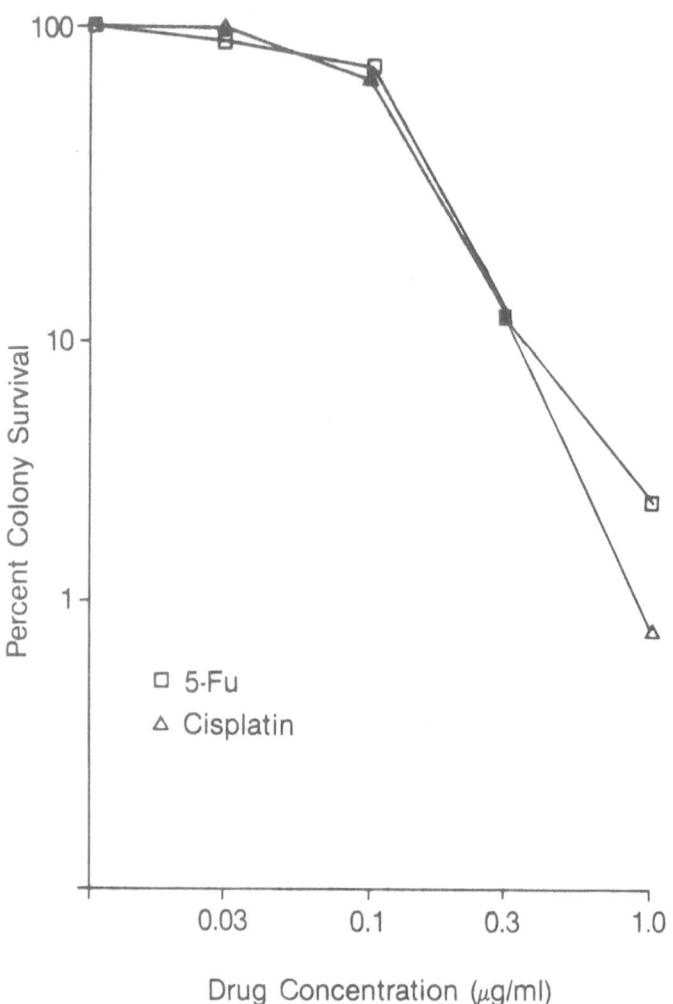

Figure 1. Sensitivity of cell line HEC–1A to 5–fluorouracil and cisplatin. With increasing concentrations of drug, decreased % colony survival is noted.

Standard chemotherapeutic agents tested with surgical specimens of endometrial cancers

At Bowman Gray School of Medicine, tumor specimens from 167 patients with uterine malignancies were processed by the laboratory for colony-forming assays. No growth was seen in 36 specimens and contamination was found in three others, precluding drug sensitivity determinations. There were, therefore, 128 specimens from which data could be obtained, 114 from solid tumors and 14 from malignant effusions. Of these specimens there were 111 that had greater than or equal to 25 colonies in each control

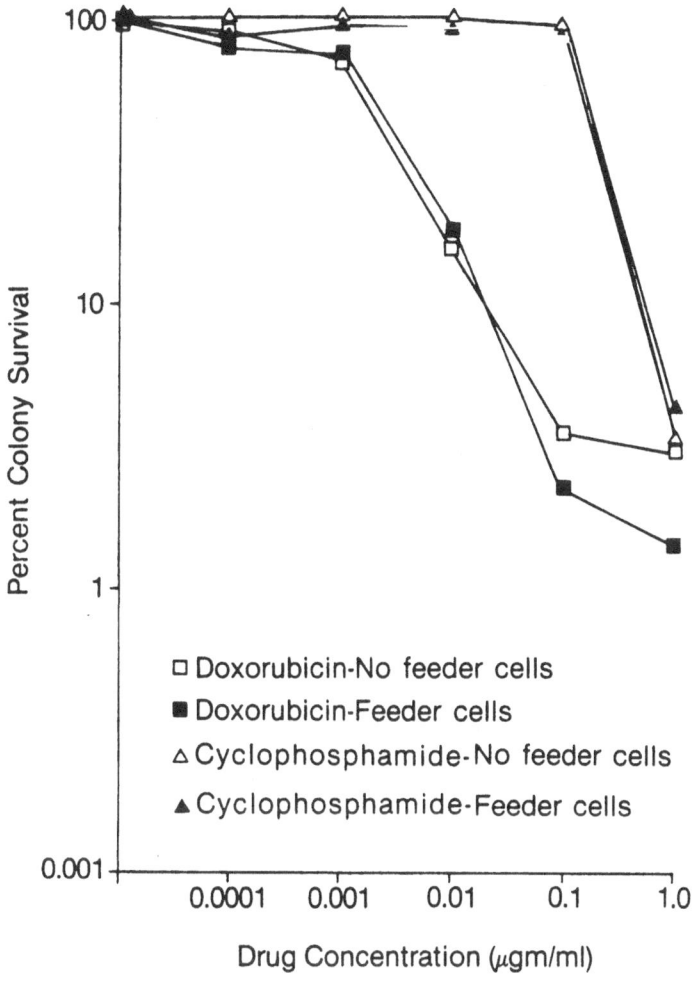

Figure 2. Sensitivity of cell line HEC–1A to doxorubicin and cyclophosphamide. Each drug has been tested with and without feeder cells. With increasing drug concentrations decreased % colony survival is noted.

culture plate and were thereby used to interpret drug sensitivity data.

Information available from colony-forming assays includes the cloning efficiency of a tumor, calculated as the ratio of colonies counted to the number of cells plated. Cloning efficiencies of solid tumors are low and expected to be in the range of 0.01% [12]. The clinically observed aggressiveness of a tumor is often related to its cloning efficiency. Histologic cell types are often correlated with cloning efficiency and are shown in Table 1. The particular uterine tumor with the highest cloning efficiency, a heterologous mixed mesodermal tumor, is also clinically one of the most aggressive. Others having an ominous clinical prognosis include the papillary serous

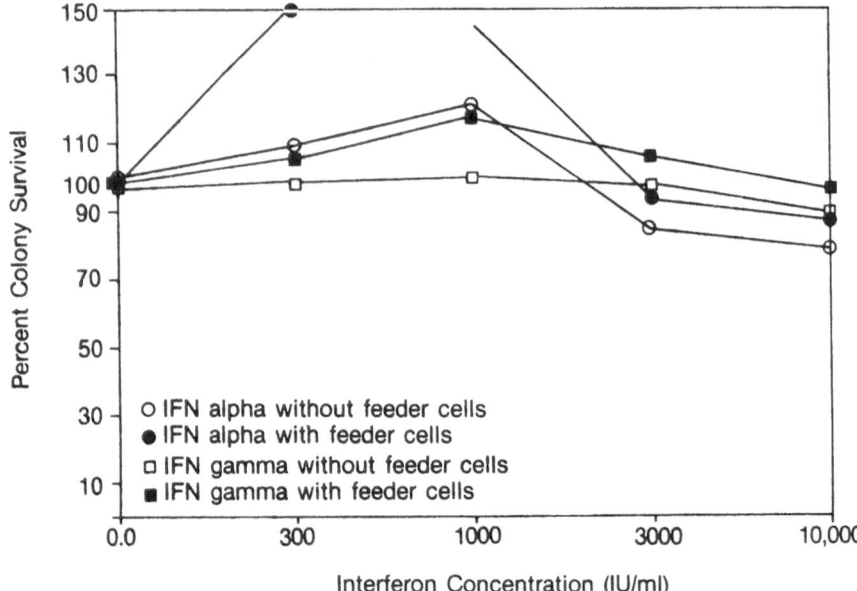

Figure 3. Sensitivity of cell line HEC–1A to interferons alpha and gamma. Each interferon is tested with and without feeder cells. With increasing concentrations, no significant decrease in colony survival is noted.

endometrial carcinoma [13] and adenosquamous carcinoma, each of which shows higher than average cloning efficiencies.

The 111 tumor specimens which grew well in culture were tested with a series of five standard chemotherapeutic agents to determine a pattern of sensitivity for endometrial cancers. Each tumor sample was tested with a peak plasma level and one-tenth peak plasma level for each drug, to the degree that the available tumor sample size permitted. The continuous exposure method, which incorporates the drug into the agarose matrix, was chosen for these studies. Antiproliferative activity of a particular drug concentration was defined as 'sensitive' when a reduction in tumor colony growth to less than 30 percent of control levels was observed. The specific activities of each of these five drugs, combining all the cell types, are shown in Table 2. A dose-related degree of response is shown by doxorubicin and cisplatin. In contrast, 5–fluorouracil shows less of a dose response, with 0.1 peak plasma level only slightly less active than a peak plasma level concentration. We can look at variations of response to drugs, separated by cell type, in Table 3. Peak plasma level concentrations, which reduce colony growth to less than 30 percent of control levels are reported showing the clinically more common cell types. The very aggressive heterologous mixed mesodermal tumor does show apparent sensitivity to three of the drugs, when 30% colony survival is determined to be the endpoint. In a clinical setting there may also be an initial partial clinical response, but the great

Table 1. Cloning efficiency of uterine cancers.

Histologic type of tumor	No. specimens	Mean cloning efficiency
Adenocarcinoma	47	0.016
Adenoacanthoma	10	0.013
Adenosquamous	14	0.022
Clear cell	2	0.006
Papillary serous	5	0.039
Mixed mesodermal — homologous	7	0.015
Mixed mesodermal — heterologous	10	0.063

Cloning efficiency expressed as ratio of colonies formed to number of cells plated.

Table 2. In vitro activity of five chemotherapeutic agents tested with uterine cancers.

Drug	Concentration	Number sensitive*/Number tested (%)
Doxorubicin	PPL	19/92 (21%)
Doxorubicin	0.1 PPL	9/76 (12%)
Cisplatin	PPL	16/95 (17%)
Cisplatin	0.1 PPL	3/71 (4%)
5–Fluorouracil	PPL	19/81 (23%)
5–Fluorouracil	0.1 PPL	12/66 (18%)
Mitomycin–C	PPL	9/61 (15%)
Mitomycin–C	0.1 PPL	6/54 (11%)
Vinblastine	PPL	2/55 (4%)
Vinblastine	0.1 PPL	1/46 (2%)

PPL = Peak plasma level.
* Sensitive = <30% colony survival.
Doxorubicin 0.6 mcg/ml; Cisplatin 2.5 mcg/ml; 5–Fluorouracil 60 mcg/ml; Mitomycin–C 0.52 mcg/ml; Vinblastine 0.783 mcg/ml.

Table 3. Percentage of specimens showing <30% colony survival related to histologic type of tumor.

Histologic type	Drugs (peak plasma level)				
	Dox	CPDD	5–FU	Mito–C	Vbl
Adenocarcinoma	19%	19%	30%	21%	4%
Adenoacanthoma	11%	13%	20%	0	0
Adenosquamous	36%	15%	36%	57%	33%
Clear cell	50%	0	0	0	0
Papillary serous	0	25%	0	0	0
Mixed mesodermal — homologous	0	0	0	0	0
Mixed mesodermal — heterologous	57%	38%	34%	0	0

Dox — doxorubicin   0.6 mcg/ml peak plasma level
CPDD — cisplatin   2.5 mcg/ml peak plasma level
5–FU — 5–fluorouracil   60 mcg/ml peak plasma level
Mito–C — mitomycin–C   0.52 mcg/ml peak plasma level
Vbl — vinblastine   0.783 mcg/ml peak plasma level.

heterogeneity of this particular tumor allows resistant subpopulations of cells to regrow following an initial response. Unfortunately, none of the drugs tested shows a high degree of in vitro activity with these patients' tumor specimens.

Investigational drugs tested with endometrial cancer specimens

At the University of Arizona in Tucson similar testing of primary endo-metrial adenocarcinoma specimens has been done, studying a wide variety of investigational drugs. Some drugs have been tested by the method of one hour exposure and others by continuous exposure. The number of speci-mens tested with the % of specimens that showed less than or equal to 30% colony survival is recorded in Table 4. Uterine sarcomas were grouped together as a separate category and were tested with two types of interferons (Table 5). Although the number of tumor samples tested with each drug is not large, there appears to be antiproliferative activity among some of the anthracycline analogues, as well as combinations of interferon gamma and tumor necrosis factor.

Application of predictive data to clinical oncology

What does it mean to a practicing oncologist to know the drug sensitivity patterns of a large group of endometrial carcinomas? Stated more specifical-ly, of what importance is drug sensitivity data in treatment planning for an individual patient? In the example of ovarian cancers, a significant experi-ence has been accumulated, correlating predictive laboratory data with response to therapy [14]. Chemotherapeutic agents that show in vitro activ-ity are correlated with 60–75% probability of a good clinical response. Conversely, in vitro resistance is correlated with greater than 90% probabil-ity of clinical nonresponse. Jones reported a group of seven patients with endometrial cancer who were given single agent chemotherapy, based upon predictive information from colony-forming assays [6]. Five patients had tumor resistance noted in vitro and showed no clinical response. One patient had sensitivity in vitro and did respond clinically. One false-positive was noted in this group, with in vitro sensitivity but in vivo resistance.

As clinicians become more experienced using many types of predictive information related to patients' responses to therapy, it is clear that no single parameter will be adequate. Host factors impact in a major way on clinical responses to therapy. In ovarian cancer, for example, performance status and the bulk of residual tumor are greater predictors of response than the laboratory data from clonogenic assays [15]. The vascular perfusion of a tumor determines whether drugs administered will ever reach tumor cells in concentrations adequate to alter growth. Heterogeneity of human tumors is

124

Table 4. Investigational drugs tested with endometrial adenocarcinomas.

Drug (peak plasma level)	Method of exposure	Number sensitive*/ Number tested (%)
4'deoxydoxorubicin	1 hour	4/12 (33%)
4'deoxydoxorubicin	Continuous	4/6 (67%)
Idarubicin	1 hour	3/12 (25%)
O–methyl–doxorubicin	Continuous	4/4 (100%)
4–demethoxy–4–epi–doxorubicin	Continuous	4/4 (100%)
4–demethoxy–daunorubicin	Continuous	3/4 (75%)
Aclacinomycin	Continuous	4/4 (100%)
Carboplatin	1 hour	1/6 (17%)
Tumor necrossis factor	Continuous	1/10 (10%)
Interferon gamma	Continuous	2/8 (25%)
Tumor necrosis factor plus interferon gamma	Continuous	3/7 (43%)
Interferon alpha	Continuous	1/4 (25%)
Tamoxifen	1 hour	1/4 (25%)
Tamoxifen	Continuous	2/15 (13%)

* Number sensitive = <30% colony survival.

Table 5. Investigational drugs tested with uterine sarcomas.

Drug (peak plasma level)	Method of exposure	Number sensitive (<30% colony survival)/Number tested (%)
Interferon alpha	Continuous	0/6 (0%)
Interferon beta	Continuous	2/4 (50%)

another reason why single agent chemotherapy will fail. Laboratory sensitivity of tumor to a particular drug is defined as colony growth reduced to less than 30% of controls. Those remaining cells that are resistant in vitro will continue to grow in the patient. Rarely will clinically achievable concentrations of a single drug reduce colony growth in vitro to less than 10% of controls, representing only a 1 log cell kill.

In order to predict more accurately the clinical outcome of any patient therapy, many parameters need to be included in a prognostic index. For endometrial cancers, important parameters include clinical stage, depth of tumor invasion of the myometrium, nuclear grade of tumor, architectural grade of tumor, proliferative activity, steroid hormone receptor levels, cloning efficiency in vitro, and chemotherapy sensitivity data. Large numbers of patients will be needed to statistically determine the degree of importance of each parameter in terms of a patient's eventual clinical outcome.

Perhaps a more significant application of available in vitro technology is the screening of new drugs for antitumor activity. By using cell lines and/or primary tumor specimens, it is possible to quickly evaluate new compounds and, thereby, to establish priorities for clinical testing of new therapies.

Clinical treatment trials for patients with uterine cancers are being conducted using many standard and investigational agents. The data presented here would suggested that long term exposure of tumor cells to 5–fluorouracil and mitomycin–C (i.e., infusion therapy regimens) would be a reasonable clinical treatment trial to propose. Other investigational compounds with notable in vitro activity are the new anthracycline analogues. Further in vitro testing of drug combinations will also yield important information that may be applied to clinical treatment protocol design.

References

1. Homesley HD, 1987. Staging and current treatments for endometrial cancer. Oncology 1:53–57.
2. Creasman WT, Morrow CP, Bundy BN, Homesley HD, Graham JE, Heller PB, 1987. Surgical pathologic spread patterns of endometrial cancer. Cancer 60:2035–2041.
3. Mittal KR, Schwartz PE, Barwick KW, 1988. Architectural grading, nuclear grading, and other prognostic indicators in Stage I endometrial adenocarcinoma with identification of high-risk and low-risk groups. Cancer 61:538–545.
4. Geisinger KR, Homesley HD, Morgan TM, Kute TE, Marshall RB, 1986. Endometrial adenocarcinoma. A multiparameter clinicopathologic analysis including the DNA profile and the sex steroid hormone receptors. Cancer 58:1518–1525.
5. Richardson GS, MacLaughlin DT, 1986. The status of receptors in the management of endometrial cancer. Clin Obstet Gynecol 29:628–637.
6. Jones CM,III, Welander CE, Berens ME, Homesley HD, 1987. In vitro growth characteristics and chemosensitivities of endometrial cancer using a soft agar clonogenic assay. Obstet Gynecol 69:237–241.
7. Shoemaker RH, Wolpert–DeFillippes MK, Kern DH, Lieber MM, Makuch RW, Melnick NR, Miller WT, Salmon SE, Simon RM, Venditti JM, Von Hoff DD, 1985. Application of a human tumor colony-forming assay to new drug screening. Cancer Res 45:2145–2153.
8. Saito T, Berens ME, Welander CE, 1986. Direct and indirect effects of human recombinant gamma interferon on tumor cells in a clonogenic assay. Cancer Res 46:1142–1147.
9. Hamburger AW, Salmon SE, 1977. Primary bioassay of human tumor stem cells. Science 197:461–463.
10. Welander CE, Morgan TM, Homesley HD, Trotta PP, Spiegel RJ, 1985. Combined recombinant human interferon alpha$_2$ and cytotoxic agents studied in the clonogenic assay. Intl J Cancer 35:721–729.
11. Kuramoto H, Tamura S, Notake Y, 1972. Establishment of a cell line of human endometrial adenocarcinoma in vitro. Am J Obstet Gynecol 114:1012–1019.
12. Steel GG, 1977. Growth kinetics of tumors. Oxford: Clarendon Press, pp. 217–267.
13. Hendrickson M, Ross J, Eifel P, Martinez A, Kempson R, 1982. Uterine papillary serous carcinoma. A highly malignant form of endometrial adenocarcinoma. Am J Surg Path 6:93–108.
14. Alberts DS, Chen HSG, Salmon SE, Surwit EA, Young L, Moon TE, Meyskens FL,Jr, 1981. Chemotherapy of ovarian cancer directed by the human tumor stem cell assay. Cancer Chemother Pharmacol 6:279–285.
15. Welander CE, 1987. Predicting response to chemotherapy with a clonogenic assay. In Ovarian Cancer — The Way Ahead (Sharp F, and Soutter WP, eds.) London: Chameleon Press Ltd. pp. 175–186.

Index

Aclacinomycin, 125
Adenoacanthoma, 29
Adenocarcinoma
  hormonal receptors in, 72
  progesterone receptors (PR)
    concentrations in, 85–87
Adenosquamous carcinoma, prognosis
  for, 28–29, 122
Adnexal metastasis
  cytology in, 44, 49
  prognosis and, 29–30
  radiotherapy for, 66, 68
Age
  at first birth, 13
  incidence and, 3–4, 13
  prognosis in surgery related to, 28
  risk factors and menarche and, 11–13
  see also Postmenopausal women;
  Premenopausal women
Alpha interferon, 119, 125
Aminothiadiazole (ATD), 103
Androstenedione, in polycystic ovary
  syndrome, 5
Anovulatory cycles, and risk factors, 6
Arterial pressure, as risk factor, 13–14
Asian women, and incidence, 3
Aziridinylbenzoquinone (AZQ), 101–102

Black women, and incidence, 2–3, 4
Bladder cancer, in staging of endometrial
  carcinoma, 26
Blood pressure, as risk factor, 13–14
Bone scan, in staging, 25–26
Breast cancer, 13
  endometrial cancer and estrogenic
    hormone treatment of, 9
  hormonal receptors in, 72
  model systems for, 74

staging of endometrial carcinoma and,
  26

CA-125 tumor marker, in staging, 26
Cancers
  endometrial cancer and estrogenic
    hormone treatment of, 9–10
  staging and presence of other, 26
  see also specific cancers
Carboplatin, 100–101, 125
Caucasian women, and incidence, 2, 4
CCNU, 102
Cervix
  prognosis and spread to, 30
  surgery for Stage II disease and, 36
Chemotherapy
  combinations in, 102, 108–111
  criteria for therapeutic effectiveness of,
    93–94
  cytotoxic drugs in, 97–103
  dose intensity analysis of, 113
  drug sensitivity tests in, 119–124
  future directions for, 114
  in vitro testing of, 117–126
  papillary serous carcinoma with, 67, 68
  rationale, 107–108
  resistance to, 111–113
  single agent, 93–104
  surgery for Stage III and IV disease
    and, 37
  see also specific agents
Chest x-ray, in staging, 25
Children, number of, as risk factor, 13
Chinese women, and incidence, 3
Chronic anovulatory syndrome, 6
Cigarette smoking, see Smoking
Cisplatin
  combination therapy with, 102, 108–
    111

127

in vitro activity of, 122
therapeutic effectiveness of, 99–100
Colon cancer, in staging of endometrial carcinoma, 26
Computerized tomography (CT), in staging, 25
Contraceptives, *see* Oral contraceptives
Curettage, in in staging, 24
Cyclophosphamide
combination therapy with, 102, 108
dose intensity analysis of, 113
sensitivity to, 119
therapeutic effectiveness of, 102–103
Cystic hyperplasia, and estrogens, 6, 7
Cytology, 41–51
depth of myometrial depth correlated with, 49
FIGO staging with, 41
incidence of malignancy in, 46–49
Indiana University–St. Vincent Hospital study of, 42–46
metastatic spread and, 44, 49
prognosis and, 30–32
recurrent disease with, 46
significance of, 41–42
surgery for Stage I disease with, 32
Cytotoxic therapy, 97–103; *see also* specific agents

Demographics, and incidence, 1–4
4′Deoxydoxorubicin, 125
DHAD, 103
Diabetes mellitus, as risk factor, 13
Dimethisterone, as risk factor, 11
Doxorubicin, 125
combination therapy with, 102, 108
in vitro activity of, 122
sensitivity to, 119
therapeutic effectiveness of, 98–99

Eastern Cooperative Oncology Group (ECOG), 102, 108
Endometrial hyperplasia
exogenous estrogens and, 6, 7, 9
incidence of endometrial cancer and, 5, 7
progestogens and, 10–11
Epidemiology, 1–15
Estradiol, as risk factor, 7–9
Estradiol dehydrogenase, 72, 78
Estrogen-induced hyperplasia

incidence of endometrial cancer and, 1, 10
progestogens in treatment of, 10
Estrogen receptors (ER)
breast tumors and, 72
frozen section documentation of, 34
nude mouse model of endometrial carcinoma and, 76, 77–78
response to progestational agents and, 96
Estrogens (endogenous)
endometrial proliferation and, 5
future directions for research on, 15
gall bladder disease and, 14
obesity and levels of, 5
progestogen supplementation of, 11
as risk factor, 5
smoking as risk factor and, 15
Estrogens (exogenous)
adenomatous endometrial hyperplasia and, 6–7
dose, as risk factor, 9
endometrial hyperplasia and, 6, 7, 9
future directions for research on, 15
incidence and, 2, 3–4, 6, 7
invasive and higher grade cancers and, 9–10
long-term effects of, 9
periodic interruption of use of, 9–10
risk factors and, 6–10
time since first use of, 7
time since last use of, 7
type used, 7–9
Estrone levels, and obesity, 5
Ethinyl estradiol, as risk factor, 7, 11
Etoposide, 103
European women, and incidence, 2–3

Fertility, and risk factors, 13
FIGO staging
cytology on, 41
drug sensitivity tests and, 117
prognosis and, 23, 25
surgery and, 23, 24–26
5-Fluorouracil, 126
in vitro activity of, 122
therapeutic effectiveness of, 103, 108
Fractional curettage, in staging, 24

Galactitol, 103
Gall bladder disease, as risk factor, 14

128

Gamma interferon, 119, 125
Genetic factors, and risk, 15
Geographic area, and incidence, 1, 2
Glucose tolerance, as risk factor, 13
Grade
   cytology correlated to, 43–44, 49
   preoperative cytology and, 54, 55
   tissue concentrations of hormonal
     receptors and, 73
Gynecologic Oncology Group (GOG), 23,
   27–30, 63, 93, 95, 97–102, 108

Hawaiian women, and incidence, 3, 4
Hexamethylmelamine, 101
Histology, and prognosis in surgery, 28–
   29
Hormone creams, as risk factor, 9
Hormone receptors, 71–90
   frozen section documentation of, 34
   prognosis in surgery and, 30–32
Hydroxylation pathway
   smoking as risk factor and, 15
   obesity and estrogen levels and, 5
Hyperplasia, *see* Estrogen-induced
   hyperplasia
Hypertension, as risk factor, 13–14
Hysterectomy
   in Stage I disease, 34–36
   in Stage II disease, 36
Hysterography, in staging, 25
Hysteroscopy, in staging, 25

ICRF-159, 103
Idarubicin, 125
Incidence
   demographic correlates of, 1–4
   estrogen replacement therapy and, 2, 3–
     4, 6, 7
   lack of endogenous progesterone and, 6
   lymph node metastasis and, 63–64
Interferons, 114
   sensitivity tests with, 119
   testing of, 125
Interleukins, 114
International Federation of Gynecologists
   and Obstetricians (FIGO), *see* FIGO
   staging
Intravenous pyelogram (IV), in staging, 25

Japanese women, and incidence, 3

Laparotomy, 32
Liver scan, in staging, 25–26
Lymph node metastasis
   cytology in, 44, 49
   incidence of, 63–64
   peritoneal metastases combined with,
     69
   radiotherapy and, 64–65, 66
   surgical technique in, 35
Lymphoma, in staging of endometrial
   carcinoma, 26

Magnetic resonance imaging (MRI), in
   staging, 25
Maori women, and incidence, 4
Medroxyprogesterone acetate (MPA), 78,
   95
Megestrol acetate, 95, 108
Menarche, and risk, 11–13
Menopause
   incidence and age of, 3–4, 13
   progesterone levels during, 6
   risk factors and, 6
   see also Postmenopausal women;
     Premenopausal women
Metastasis
   CA-125 tumor marker in, 26
   cytology in, 44, 49
   progestin therapy response rate in, 71
   as prognostic factor, 29
   surgical technique in, 35, 37
   see also Adnexal metastasis; Lymph
     node metastasis
Methotrexate, 103
Methyl CCNU, 102
Methyl-doxorubicin, 125
MGBG, 102
Mitomycin-C, 123, 126
Mitoxantrone, 103
Model systems for endometrial carcinoma
   development of, 74–77
   treatment evaluations with, 78–80
Monoclonal antibodies against
   progesterone
   receptors (PR), 80–83
Mucinous adenocarcinoma, 29
Myometrial invasion
   cytology correlated with, 49
   lymph node metastasis and, 64
   preoperative radiotherapy and, 54, 56,
     57
   as prognostic factor, 29

Nationality, and and incidence, 2–3
Nitrosoureas, 102
Nodal metastasis, *see* Lymph node
    metastasis
Norethindrone, and endometrial
    hyperplasia, 10
North Central Cancer Treatment Group
    (NCCTG), 100
Nulliparity, as risk factor, 13

Obesity
    estrogen levels and, 5
    progesterone levels and, 6
    risk factors with, 5, 6
O-methyl-doxorubicin, 125
Oracon, as risk factor, 11
Oral contraceptives (OCs), as risk factor,
    11
Ovarian cancer
    genetic factors in, 15
    incidence of endometrial cancer and, 5
    staging of endometrial carcinoma and,
    26

Papillary serous carcinoma
    chemotherapy testing with, 121–122
    histology of, 29
    radiotherapy for, 67, 68
Pelvis
    cytology and metastatic spread to, 46,
    49
    radiation exposure in, as risk factor, 14
    staging and ultrasound of, 26
Percutaneous estradiol, 7–9
Peritoneal cytology of, *see* Cytology
Peritoneal metastases
    lymph node metastases combined with,
    69
    prognosis and, 29–30
    radiotherapy for, 66, 68
1-Phenylalanine mustard, 108
Physical examination, in staging, 24
Piperazinedione, 103
Polycystic ovaries
    estrogen levels in, 5
    incidence of endometrial cancer and, 5,
    6
    lack of endogenous progesterone and, 6
Postmenopausal women
    cigarette smoking as risk factor in, 14–
    15

    obesity and estrogen levels in, 5
    progestogen supplementation in, 11
    prognosis in surgery for, 28
Premenopausal women
    cigarette smoking as risk factor in, 14–
    15
    incidence in, 6
    prognosis in surgery for, 28
Progesterone
    anovulatory cycles and, 6
    cytology and, 45
    polycystic ovary syndrome and, 6
    risk factors and lack of endogenous, 6
Progesterone receptors (PR), 71
    breast tumors and, 72
    frozen section documentation of, 34
    monoclonal antibodies against, 80–83
    response rate to, 71, 96
    tissue concentrations of, 72, 73–74, 83–
    88
Progestin
    criteria for therapeutic effectiveness of,
    95–96
    nude mouse model of endometrial
    carcinoma and evaluation of, 77–78
    response rate to, 71
    tamoxifen therapy combined with, 78–
    80
    tests of sensitivity to, 72–73
Progestogens
    future directions for research on, 15
    risk factors and lack of, 10–11
Prognosis
    adnexal and intraperitoneal spread and,
    29–30
    age and menopausal stage as, 28
    cervical involvement and, 33
    FIGO staging and, 23, 25
    histology and, 28–29
    hormone receptors ad, 30–32
    myometrial invasion and, 29
    surgery and, 27–32
    uterine size as, 28

Race, and and incidence, 2–3, 4
Radionuclide scanning, in staging, 25–26
Radiotherapy
    adnexal metastases and, 66, 68
    combination of nodal and peritoneal
    metastases and, 69
    high-dose versus low-dose, 58